THE POWER OF POSTPARTUM SELF-CARE AND RECOVERY

PRACTICAL STRATEGIES TO REJUVENATE YOUR BODY, NURTURE YOUR MIND, NAVIGATE DEPRESSION, MANAGE FATIGUE, AND FIND CONFIDENCE IN MOTHERHOOD

JOCELYN BRABYN HUNTER

TABLE OF CONTENTS

INTRODUCTION

"The moment a child is born, the mother is also born. She never existed before. The woman existed, but the mother, never. A mother is something absolutely new." [1]

BHAGWAN SHREE RAJNEESH

I had just completed 24 hours of excruciating labor, and I was at last resting in the recovery room of the hospital where my first child had been born. As I held my infant daughter, my heart was already swelling larger than I had ever thought possible. While I gazed at her sleeping, angelic face, a nurse was briefing me on how to care for my newborn. I smiled and nodded as I let her words wash over my exhausted, sleep-deprived brain until I heard the words that made me look up at her, not sure I'd heard correctly.

"You want me to wake her up every four hours . . . to feed her?"

"Yes."

"So I have to wake up every four hours in order to wake her up?"

"Yes, we don't want her to get dehydrated. Babies can sleep so soundly that they might not wake up even if they need more milk."

My head spun at the implications. I had already gone more than 48 hours without sleep. Would I set an alarm then, every four hours, disrupting my own hard-earned sleep? How could this nurse ask that of me after everything I had been through to bring this baby into the world? Didn't she care about my needs?

And just like that, it hit me—this was my new reality.

My own need for sleep was no longer the top priority—my top priority had become the tiny, fragile being in my arms: keeping her alive, keeping her safe, and making her feel loved. And just like that, my life was changed forever, just like yours will soon be if it hasn't already.

Becoming a mother is one of the most empowering and intense experiences a woman can undergo. It feels like everything changes in an instant, and you're reborn into a role filled with unconditional love, deep responsibility, and a new set of challenges. A new mother will feel the fullest range of emotions from the purest joy to the lowest moments of self-doubt. When you become a mother, the love you feel for your child is immeasurable. Still, the weight of so much responsibility can be crippling.

If you're anything like me, you'll be questioning everything in the early days; How do you keep your baby healthy? How do you find time to care for yourself? How could you possibly balance your own needs with those of your newborn? I kept myself awake during many sleepless nights, asking myself these questions. I felt anxious and inadequate, leading to restlessness and emotional instability, all while suffering from the physical discomfort of postpartum recovery.

Within the community of new mothers, you're not alone in feeling lost, exhausted, and unsure of how to move forward. I have struggled to balance the same mix of joy and dread that comes with holding your newborn for the first time, and I've felt the crushing fatigue that follows the exhilaration of being a mother. There's constant pressure to be a perfect mother, flawlessly avoiding any possible mistake. News flash: we're all messing up a little bit, at least some of the time. Regardless, we all are deserving of help and support, and there is no shame in seeking it.

As someone who's experienced what you're going through, my goal is to pass my insights on, offering you support on your path to physical recovery. This book will teach you to set boundaries with loved ones, rekindle lost intimacy with a partner, and consistently strengthen the bond you have with your baby.

My writing will give you the opportunity to process your emotions and maintain a positive mindset by providing you with guided journaling prompts and affirmations that reduce your feelings of insecurity and bring forward self-trust. Every new mom has the potential to approach each day with confidence in their ability to remain resilient and connected to their child, all with the peace of mind that they're capable of handling whatever's coming.

As an anthropologist and a researcher, I've felt compelled to study how various cultures navigate the complexities of postpartum recovery in preparation for writing this book. However, even more importantly, I've lived them. I have been through the highs and lows of childbirth with two home births and one hospital birth with the support of a doula. There are a few things that have risen above everything else during my mission to be a secure mother: self-care, resilience, and community.

You don't have to struggle through the challenges of new motherhood alone, even when it feels like it. Let this book serve as a reminder of the validity of your feelings and the potential you have to be a positive and impactful figure to your children. I aim to provide a source of comfort and empowerment, acknowledging your feelings and challenges and guiding you to reclaim your joyful strength.

You're on the right path. Take a deep breath, and get ready to explore the complexities of motherhood from a voice that truly understands you.

CHAPTER ONE

WHY IS POSTPARTUM SELF-CARE IMPORTANT?

"You are worth the quiet moment. You are worth the deeper breaths and the time it takes to slow down, be still, and rest." [1]

MORGAN HARPER NICHOLS

These words serve as a powerful reminder: Amidst all the demands of caring for a newborn, your mind and body don't just stop needing care. Your well-being is deserving of your attention, even when you're consumed by the needs of your baby. In these crucial moments, taking time to slow down, breathe, and rest might feel like a luxury, but it's a necessity for your happiness and that of your family. Giving yourself a break probably doesn't hang out at the top of your priority list when you're caring for your newborn. Ignoring your own health completely, however, significantly impedes your ability to care for your baby as best as possible.

Welcome to your "fourth trimester." While not discussed as often, this time offers unique opportunities for growth and inspiration, for you and your baby alike. You've made it through the transformative process of pregnancy and childbirth, and a complete rebirth has taken place for you; You're no longer just an individual, but a creator of life. You and your baby have a deep connection that feels natural, but navigating the world with new responsibilities sometimes does not.

The fourth trimester begins as soon as your baby is born, and it ends 90 days later. This term was coined by Dr. Harvey Karp in 2002 to describe the time period when a new mother adjusts to her role as a parent while her newborn adjusts to being outside of the womb. This unique time is full of significant physical and emotional changes for both the mother and the baby. The baby is experiencing an environment vastly different from the warm, snug uterus, and the mother is easing into a period of physical recovery, adaptation, and lifelong bonding with the newborn.[2]

While this moment often feels more like a rebirth, the fourth trimester is named that way to reflect its importance; your baby is still in a phase of development that closely resembles the experiences they had in utero. During this time, babies benefit from practices that recreate the conditions of the womb, like gentle rocking, soothing sounds, and warmth, helping them feel secure and supported in their gradual adjustment to the world around them.

Your fourth trimester will be rich with challenges and opportunities. Pregnancy and childbirth are followed by a long period of recovery, as your organs shift back into place, your hormones fluctuate, and you navigate the physical demands of breastfeeding.[3] It's not unlikely that you would feel exhaustion, discomfort, and emotional turmoil during this time period, all while trying to balance it with helping your child adjust to a new environment, feed, and develop trust in the new world.

Taking care of yourself is an essential part of leading a fulfilling and healthy life, but the need for self-care escalates after child-birth. Postpartum self-care refers to the intentional actions and practices a new mother engages in to take care of her physical, mental, and emotional health by engaging in activities that bring a sense of joy, relaxation, or peace. These little actions have an immense impact on the well-being of the parent and, as a result, the relationship they have with their child. Despite this, self-care is often neglected by new mothers, who may feel the need to sacrifice all of their time or energy for their newborn.

Many of us have been taught that being a good mom requires putting our children's needs above all else, even at the expense of our own well-being. These messages have been sent explicitly and implicitly, through external societal voices and the opinions of those close to us. With this expectation, so many mothers feel that their own needs should be last on their priority list if it even makes the cut. Even when we need it most, it almost feels selfish to take care of ourselves, relax, or decompress physically and mentally. This is especially true when we need to first meet the demands of caring for someone who is completely dependent on us.

What many of us fail to realize, however, is how truly necessary self-care is for mothers and their children to succeed. If a mom is constantly giving without taking time to replenish her own energy, she is likely to reach a severe burnout period. It may manifest in her as physical exhaustion, heightened stress, and postpartum depression. A mother suffering from burnout has a significantly harder time caring for her child with stability and confidence.

Just like it was during pregnancy, anything that has an effect on you is likely to have an impact on your baby, too. When a mother neglects her own physical and mental health, her exhaustion and overwhelm can impair her ability to properly bond with the child. Your fourth trimester is a critical point in your child's life, where you need to make sure you're forming a balanced attachment with them, responding to their needs properly, and providing a nurturing presence that will make up their emotional foundation going forward.

Have you ever heard that you're supposed to put your own oxygen mask on before helping others on an airplane? If an emergency occurs, you need to breathe in order to stay conscious long enough to help those around you. This principle remains true in the context of parenting; If you're balanced and full of life, your child is likely to mirror this. If you're tired and cranky, your baby will likely be the same (if not worse!)

There's a lot of change in your fourth trimester, and with it comes new challenges, too. Self-care has the ability to reduce some of the weight of these difficulties, allowing you to navigate the transition into motherhood more smoothly. It sometimes seems a bit luxurious, but the main goal of self-care is to keep fatigue at bay and prevent more severe issues like depression or heightened anxiety.[4] Just like your child, you need the appropriate care and attention to support your health and recovery. In turn, these efforts will create a more stable and nurturing environment for your family.

Feelings of depression and insecurity can become enlarged when you're constantly surrounded by the common myths forced upon motherhood. It seems like everyone has something to say about how a mother should look, act, and behave after having a baby. There are numerous unrealistic expectations forced onto new mothers, leading to misunderstandings about what is "normal" during the recovery phase. This pressure can have disastrous effects on a mother's physical and emotional well-being. Let's address some of the most common myths and misconceptions related to the postpartum period:

Myth: If you don't have any concerning symptoms, you don't need to follow up with your doctor.

Fact: Even if you're feeling fine, you need to attend all scheduled and recommended check-ups after childbirth. Many issues don't present as obvious issues; high blood pressure, infections, and mental health concerns can sneak up on new mothers. These appointments keep you and your healthcare provider updated on your recovery process so you can adjust anything or address underlying issues that might have an impact on your long-term health.[5]

Myth: You will immediately bounce back to your pre-baby weight, and if you don't, you're doing something wrong.

Fact: The idea that a mother needs to "bounce back" to her pre-baby body is unnecessary and irrational. Childbirth is an incredible feat that puts an immense amount of pressure on a woman's body, and it's completely natural to see changes in your weight, body shape, or jean size.[6] It's hard to even think about weight loss when you're so focused on physical recovery, healing, bonding, and nurturing your mental space. Embrace the changes in your body, as well as where they came from, and prioritize health and strength as you recover.

Myth: At 6 weeks postpartum, you're pretty much completely healed and ready for anything.

Fact: While your doctor may clear you for certain activities at the 6-week mark, making a full recovery can take significantly longer. Your body will continue to heal and adjust for months following this point, so easing into strenuous activities is advised. Most importantly, every mother has a unique recovery timeline, so be sure to actively listen to your body and not rush the healing process.

Myth: Leaking, prolapse, painful sex, and other pelvic floor issues are just things you have to live with after having a baby.

Fact: While these conditions are common after childbirth, you don't have to live with them. If you're suffering from issues with incontinence, pelvic organ prolapse, or pain during sex, you should address your concerns with a healthcare provider. In many cases, they'll suggest physical therapy or other treatments that intend to help you recover and live a higher quality of life.

Myth: You're a bad parent if you don't [. . .]

Fact: There is no single "right" way to parent, and constantly trying to find one creates irrational guilt and pressure. Being a mother is not one-size-fits-all; each parent and child is unique, and what works for them might not work for another family. If you have faith in your abilities and instincts and do what's best for your situation, you're doing what you need to do to be a good parent.

Myth: The baby bump disappears after the child is born.

Fact: After childbirth, it's pretty normal for a belly to remain enlarged for a while. Your entire body is adjusted in order to properly support the growth of the fetus, so your uterus, muscles, and skin all need some time to shrink back to their original form. This doesn't happen overnight. A postpartum body is a testament to all of the miracles it performed; it's normal for it to take weeks or even months to return to a "normal" state.

Myth: Everyone gets postpartum depression. It's not a big deal.

Fact: Not every new mother will experience postpartum depression. However, it is a serious condition that affects many new mothers, and it can have a large effect on a mother's ability to raise her children properly if it goes unacknowledged. While many mothers suffer from short-term feelings of sadness or irritability after giving birth, postpartum depression is found in those who struggle with intense, persistent feelings of sadness, hopelessness, and guilt, as well as physical symptoms like aches and pains. Never discount your overwhelmingly negative feelings as "normal"; your mental health should always be taken seriously.

Being able to recognize all of the misconceptions associated with the postpartum period can help you slash through all the negativity and approach yourself with more compassion and understanding as you move through your own recovery process. When you're in your fourth trimester, the primary requirement is finding a path that supports you and your baby's health and well-being.

Everyone's life looks a little different after childbirth. There are postpartum recovery traditions deeply rooted in a variety of cultures, each full of beliefs and activities that have been passed down for centuries. These traditions often emphasize support, rest, and nutrition, reflecting the need to care for a mother as she recovers from childbirth.

In South Korea, the postpartum period is referred to as *Sanhujori,* and it mostly includes consuming healthy foods and doing light exercises that warm up the body. While some mothers spend three weeks to a month in a care center, others simply remain in their homes and focus on rest, warmth, and nutrition. Caretakers often provide recovering mothers with nutrient-rich foods like seaweed soup to help replenish the nourishment lost during childbirth.[7]

In Mexico, mothers are expected to rest for 40 days after giving birth during a period called *La Cuarentena.* Most moms refrain from housework and sexual activities during this time, and other family members will chip in to help with chores and cooking.

In Chinese tradition, mothers spend the first 30 to 40 days after childbirth in strict confinement, where they avoid going outside, bathing, or engaging in physical activity. This practice is referred to as *Zuo Yue Zi,* or "sitting the month," and it focuses mostly on staying warm and eating nourishing foods to restore energy and balance.

In Iceland, the government's social welfare system strongly supports mothers, and they are able to receive regular visits from midwives who monitor their recovery and provide guidance on early baby care. There's an emphasis on providing support to mothers, making sure they are not isolated from family and community members. Stable mental health is an essential part of a mother's recovery.

In Nigeria, a new mom's mother or MIL will come to stay with the new family for the first 40 days, where she'll care for the baby and the household. This tradition is known as *Omugwo*, and it allows the new mother to have a moment to focus completely on recovery. She'll often be given herbal baths and a monitored diet to regain her strength and health.

In India, *Ayurveda* was invented over 5,000 years ago, offering a system of medicine that takes a holistic approach to postpartum care based on the idea that the body, mind, and spirit are inherently connected. Balancing these elements is the key to maintaining health and well-being during the recovery. Ayurveda has a long history rooted in the Vedic culture in India. The word itself means "the science of life," and it encompasses various aspects of health like diet, lifestyle, and spiritual practices to support a new mother. This practice, while ancient, is still widely used now, as more people are seeking holistic approaches to their health.[8]

Like other cultures, Ayurveda places a strong emphasis on the use of herbs to strengthen the body and improve digestion and milk production. Herbal preparations are tailored to each mother's *dosha* and can include ashwagandha, shatavari, and turmeric.

Gentle yoga practices are often encouraged in Ayurveda, as they can help new mothers regain their strength, flexibility, and mental clarity. After childbirth, new mothers should focus on yoga poses that support the core, pelvic floor, and back, as these areas are particularly impacted by pregnancy. Meditation is also commonly used and provides a workout of the mind. In Ayurvedic postpartum care, new mothers use meditation or deep breathing exercises to reduce stress, calm their thoughts, and provide a sense of emotional balance amid the emotional challenges of that fourth trimester.

Ayurveda also offers a variety of purification practices to help cleanse the body of toxins and restore a sense of balance. There are gentle detoxification methods like warm oil massages and steam baths, and there are more intensive sessions that also fit into healing and rejuvenation efforts. Counseling is also provided and is considered an important aspect of the postpartum process. New mothers need emotional support and benefit from guidance while integrating the physical, mental, and spiritual changes that come with motherhood.

Many cultures acknowledge the value of a gentle and stable postpartum recovery, and they provide comprehensive, individualized plans that address the unique needs of each new mother. You can do a bit of research to find what works best for you, but the primary goal should be to find balance, nourishment, and emotional support throughout the fourth trimester.

As you may have noticed already, it's easy to lose sight of your own needs while you're caring for a newborn. While it feels like you've made a commitment to your child to give them your full attention, it's equally important to make that same commitment to yourself. Consider engaging in a self-care pledge, using your words to promise that you'll continue to offer yourself the same kindness, compassion, and care that you give to your child. By making this commitment, you're acknowledging the importance of your own well-being and its effect on how you care for your baby. Here are a few self-care pledges you can carry with you as you continue through your recovery process:

- I will listen to my body's needs.
- I will give myself the time I need to rest, recover, and heal.

- I will nourish my body with healthy, nutrient-rich foods that support my postpartum health.
- I will practice kindness toward myself and let go of unrealistic expectations.
- I will embrace the changes I see in my body.
- I will seek support when I need it.
- I will make time for activities that bring me a sense of joy or peace.
- I will remind myself that I am the best mother I can be.
- I will make time for self-care, and I will remind myself that it is not selfish.
- I will protect my mental health with boundaries and emotional acknowledgment.

With each pledge you proclaim, you're making a powerful statement that your own well-being is worth the time and effort. Committing to self-care is an ongoing process that evolves as you do.

The fourth trimester of your pregnancy is a period of adjustment that is just as crucial as the previous ones. The significance of this time and its ability to affect you and your baby cannot be understated. If you continue to acknowledge and grow from the challenges you face and prioritize your self-care, you'll lay a foundation for a smooth recovery and a powerful bond with your child. I encourage you to use the self-care pledge as a way to kick off your recovery process and begin navigating the ups and downs of early motherhood with greater confidence.

We'll next go over the physical changes that your body undergoes after giving birth, offering you an empowering approach to postpartum recovery that focuses on nurturing you and the baby.

CHAPTER TWO

EMBRACING YOUR BODY'S JOURNEY

"I think a woman's body after having a baby is pretty amazing . . . you just did the most incredible miracle that life has to offer. I mean, you gave birth to a human being!" [1]

BLAKE LIVELY

These words capture a truth that is easy to forget amid postpartum changes: your body has accomplished something amazing. Nurturing and bringing forth life is a feat that deserves infinite recognition and celebration, but for many mothers, this time is plagued with challenges surrounding body image. Of course, when you grow a human inside of your body, a few changes accompany it: stretch marks, weight fluctuations, and loose skin. These are completely normal, but they can lead to feelings of insecurity and dissatisfaction. These overwhelming feelings make it hard to recall the incredible voyage your body has taken.

Your fourth trimester is marked by a variety of physical changes as your body starts the recovery process following childbirth. Many share these changes as a natural part of healing, but they often come as an uncomfortable surprise. Having an understanding of what to expect can help you deal with the common physical changes that may occur with greater confidence and self-compassion. Let's take a look at some of these bodily changes:

- **Incisional Drainage:** If you had a cesarean section (C-section) or an episiotomy, you may experience drainage from the incision site as it heals. This will look like clear or blood-tinged fluid.
- **Breast Discharge and Engorgement:** Following childbirth, your breasts will begin producing a nutrient-rich "pre-milk" called colostrum. This fluid is essential for your baby's feeding. You may notice that your breasts become swollen, hard, and painful, and they may even release discharge in the form of colostrum, milk, or a small amount of blood.
- **Discomfort in the Perineal Area:** The perineum is the area between the vagina and the anus. This area often experiences significant strain during a vaginal delivery, so it's common to feel discomfort or pain in this area as it heals. Try using cold packs or warm packs in this area to relieve some of the pain.
- **Uterine Contractions:** After birth, your uterus will begin the process of contracting back to its pre-pregnancy size. This can take several weeks and often brings contractions known as "afterpains" that feel like menstrual cramps. These pains are usually the strongest during breastfeeding, as they prompt the release of oxytocin, a hormone that aids in the contraction.

- **Urination Contractions and Incontinence:** You may experience contractions in your bladder or difficulty controlling your urine flow following childbirth. This is known as urinary incontinence, and it occurs as a result of the strain that birth puts on the muscles of your pelvic floor. Like any muscle, they need time to regain their strength.[2]

- **Constipation:** It's common to be constipated after childbirth, especially if you're taking pain medication or recovering from a C-section. There are a variety of things that may be contributing to this issue: hormonal changes, reduced physical activity, and the pressure of the uterus on the intestines. Constipation can be addressed in a variety of ways: eating fiber-dense foods, taking stool softeners, and staying hydrated.

- **Excessive Perspiration:** Postpartum sweating is a common way for postpartum bodies to get rid of the extra fluids they retain during pregnancy. This is common at night, and while it may be uncomfortable, it's generally not a cause for concern. Opt for lightweight clothing and keep your bedroom cool to manage night sweats.

- **Separated Stomach Muscles:** A uterus that grows during pregnancy may cause the rectus abdominis muscles (AKA your six-pack) to separate. This is a condition known as diastasis recti, and it can lead to a bulge in the middle of the abdomen that becomes visible when you strain or contract your muscles.[3]

- **Skin Pigmentation Changes:** Hormonal inconsistencies during pregnancy can lead to skin pigmentation changes, like darkening on the face (melasma) and around the abdomen (linea nigra). These pigmentation changes often fade over time, but they may not disappear entirely. Just like other skin pigmentation, using gentle skin care products and protecting your skin from the sun can help manage this change.

- **Anemia:** During delivery, the blood loss can often lead to anemia. This is characterized by fatigue, weakness, and pale skin. Anemia is treated with iron supplements and iron-rich foods, like lean meats, leafy greens, and fortified cereals.

- **Back Pain:** You may have noticed that the physical strain of carrying a baby and going through labor can leave you with lingering back pain. This can be worsened by poor posture during breastfeeding or simply carrying your newborn in your arms. This can be combated with gentle stretching, physical therapy, and generally maintaining mindfulness of your posture.

- **Vaginal Changes:** It's normal to experience changes in the appearance and feel of your vaginal following a delivery. The tissues may be swollen and tender, and it may feel generally looser than before your pregnancy.

- **Stretch Marks:** Stretch marks are extremely common in the postpartum period, and they often appear as reddish or purple streaks that fade to a lighter color. Pregnancy causes your skin to stretch rapidly, causing these visible tiger stripes. Keeping your skin moisturized and using effective skincare can help reduce their appearance.

- **Hair Loss:** Losing hair in your postpartum period is a common occurrence as your hormone levels adjust following labor. For many women, a noticeable shedding of hair occurs around three to six months after giving birth.[4] This is usually temporary, but it can be particularly distressing. A balanced diet and gentle hair care can help your hair return to its normal growth cycle.

These changes can be a bit distressing at first, but they are a testament to the incredible feats your body has achieved. With that being said, caring for your body is absolutely crucial during this time to maintain your overall health and to make sure the healing process runs smoothly. There are a variety of ways to go about this, but it's important to keep in mind that your breasts and vagina require a bit of special attention. They've gone through significant changes from pregnancy and childbirth, so caring for them properly will help you have a more comfortable fourth trimester with fewer complications overall.

Let's get real about changes. As a woman, you probably sigh wearily at the thought of going bra shopping. I get it; it's tedious, and it seems like the cycle of needing a new one is never-ending. However, if there's ever been a time when you've needed a supportive bra the most, it's during the time following a pregnancy. Wearing a well-fitting and supportive bra can help manage some of the changes in your breast size, helping you reduce discomfort. Go ahead and push that bra that's two sizes too small to the back of the drawer; Anything too tight is likely to restrict milk flow and can lead to clogged ducts and even mastitis. You'll want something soft and breathable, possibly with adjustable straps for easy access.[5]

The skin on your breasts may become dry or irritated when you're nursing or using a pump. This is normal, but it doesn't have to be. With consistent use of a gentle, unscented moisturizer, you'll find a bit of relief.

This might be the first time you've ever considered caring for your nipples as a part of your routine, but it's pretty important for breastfeeding mothers. Irritated nipples can become cracked and dry. Lanolin or a similar nipple cream can help with this pain, and allowing your nipples to air dry after breastfeeding can also make a significant difference. Some midwives recommend expressing a drop of milk after nursing and gently spreading it on the nipple to prevent dryness, and this is a technique I used most often. These strategies can help, but if you're experiencing persistent or intense nipple pain, be sure to consult a healthcare provider or lactation consultant.[6]

Some mothers are eager to smoke after nine months without the ability to do so. As tempting as it may be, try to refrain from it. Smoking can impair your circulation and increase the risk of infections like mastitis, which can have painful and long-term implications on your overall health. Quitting is often easier said than done; if you're really struggling, try seeking support from peers or professionals.

Your breasts may not look or feel the same way they did before pregnancy, and that's totally okay. I can recall staring in the mirror, at what looked to me to be misshapen lumps where my breasts used to be, and feeling dreadful. This is normal. Your breasts play a major role in carrying and nursing a child, so be sure to thank them for their support and embrace the changes as a part of your body's ability to care for a little human.

Some breast tenderness and lumps may just be indications of clogged milk ducts, a common occurrence during breastfeeding. However, you will want to closely monitor your breasts during this time for any unusual lumps, persistent pain, or redness, which may be signs of a mastitis infection.

Obviously, your vagina and perineum are the other major players in the childbirth game. Your vagina undergoes significant changes during a vaginal delivery, and proper care is essential for relieving some of the challenges that occur as a result.

Good hygiene is the enemy of infections. If you've had a tear or episiotomy during delivery, you'll want to give special attention to the perineum area. Use warm water and mild, unscented soap to gently clean the area on a daily basis. After using the bathroom, wipe only from front to back to prevent bacteria from spreading from the rectal area.

After labor, you'll experience postpartum bleeding for a few weeks or so. This is referred to as lochia, and many women use pads the same way they would during a menstrual period. When using a pad, be sure to change its frequency to stay clean and reduce any risk of infection. Refrain from using tampons, as they're more likely to introduce bacteria.

A squirt bottle, or peri bottle, can be extremely helpful for keeping the perineal area clean when wiping feels a bit uncomfortable. It's a bit like using a bidet: Fill a squirt bottle with warm water—even better, add a bit of Epsom salt or make an herbal sitz bath tea--and gently squirt it over your perineum after using the bathroom or during daily cleaning. This can soothe the area and protect you from irritation. If you had a vaginal birth, I cannot emphasize enough how helpful it is to use the peri bottle when you have your first bowel movement after delivery! The warm water really helps to soothe any pain or discomfort you might feel during the movement.

I probably don't have to do too much work to convince you to take a warm, soothing bath. Soaking in a warm bath or sitz bath can help reduce perineal pain and promote both physical and emotional healing. Adding a bit of Epsom salt, baking soda, or brewed sitz bath herbs to the water can help you prevent swelling and aid in cleaning the area. Just be sure it's not too hot; steaming water can make the area even more irritated than before, as can harsh soaps or additives like bubble bath.

A perineal massage can be extremely helpful for relieving discomfort, especially if you've experienced a vaginal tear or episiotomy. You can start gently massaging in this area after the initial healing phase, typically after a few weeks.

Your body needs a lot of time to heal after childbirth. Unfortunately, this means avoiding inserting anything into the vagina, like using tampons or engaging in sexual intercourse, for at least six weeks. Most of the time, your healthcare provider can help you figure out when you're all-clear. When you're still healing, vaginal insertion may lead to increased pain or further infection in the perineal area.

Many mothers had a cesarean section and had to go through the healing process for an incision rather than for the perineum. As with any wound, you'll need to give this area special attention. Keep the incision clean using mild soap and water, and only dry it by patting it gently with a towel. You won't want to rub your incision too harshly. Tight clothing can cause irritation and discomfort, so try to opt for loose, breathable clothing as much as possible. Follow your healthcare provider's advice regarding the removal of any staples or stitches present in your incision. They are usually removed within a week or two after delivery, but it depends on how the healing process is going. The fourth trimester is a crucial time for healing; monitor your incision closely, looking for any signs of infection like increased redness, swelling, warmth, or discharge. If you notice any irregularities, contact your healthcare provider immediately.

If you've just delivered a child, your body has gone through a lot in the last year. Each little section of your body deserves special attention and care, including your mind. Pregnancy and labor can be just as tough on our mental health, and the leading cause of this is often a lowered sense of self-esteem due to bodily changes. Many people, including yourself, may be expecting your body to just magically "bounce back" to its pre-pregnancy state after giving birth. This idea is pervasive and simply incorrect, often fueled by unrealistic societal expectations and media portrayal of postpartum celebrity or influencer bodies. Worrying about what your body looks like and comparing it to others (or your own) doesn't help you heal, and feelings of inadequacy can make it hard to adequately care for yourself during this time. With this in mind, one of your top priorities should be to approach yourself with kindness and patience. You've heard this before, but your body has just undergone an incredible transformation.

It's obvious that pregnancy affects your weight, skin elasticity, and muscle tone. However, when these changes become visible, it can still be quite shocking and distressing. Women have a built-in fear of stretch marks, loose skin, or any other physical changes that are often looked down on in society. A negative body image doesn't just stay in your head; it spills over into your relationships, mental health, and overall quality of life. Some mothers even feel an unavoidable sense of resentment toward their newborns as their brain tries to account for all the extra weight.

Here's a reality check: Weight gained during pregnancy doesn't disappear immediately after birth. It might take several months, or even years, to lose the weight. This is completely normal—your body has been through likely one of the most significant events of your life, and it deserves time to heal and adjust.

Every woman's body is unique, like a snowflake. What happens to one mama won't necessarily happen to you, so making any kind of comparison is a waste of your time. We've all fallen into the trap of scrolling some random girl's social media page and taking mental notes of all the things she may have that you don't, or vice versa. *I cannot stress how much you should avoid doing this enough.* Most bodily changes are unavoidable, and there are some things you won't be able to change about the way you look. What's important is learning to love what you've got. Focus on your own path and search for daily appreciation of the individuality of your body.

Mark Twain once said that "comparison is the death of joy,"[7] and this reigns even more true in the modern world of social media. Never, *ever*, compare yourself to celebrities or influencers who appear to bounce back in mere weeks after childbirth. No matter how real it seems, these posts are not reflections of reality. Many of the women who seem to lose all the weight after labor have access to personal trainers, nutritionists, photo editing resources, or other support that most new mothers don't have. Trying to attain an unrealistic standard will leave you running in circles, searching for perfection that doesn't exist.

When many of us see weight gain, our first thought is to book it to the gym. Exercise is extremely beneficial for your physical and mental health, but after childbirth, you should never push yourself too soon or too hard. Consult with your obstetrician before beginning a new exercise regimen. They'll likely recommend starting with gentle activities, like stretches, bends, or walking. As your body heals, you'll be able to safely and gradually increase your activity level.

With so many bodily changes, it's normal to feel a bit down about your appearance. While you probably look just as beautiful as ever, you can carve out a bit of time for self-care to enhance the feelings of self-love that may not be coming as naturally after birth. Treat yourself to a new hairstyle, get a cute manicure, or do a shopping spree for some well-fitting clothes that make you feel good. Implementing small acts of self-care into your daily life can boost your confidence long-term and help bring out some positive feelings regarding your appearance.

It can be hard to be constantly striving to love every single aspect of your body, especially during the postpartum period. To lift some of this pressure off, aim for body neutrality. This concept includes accepting your body as it is without any judgment. Constant positivity can be exhausting. Sometimes all you have to do is recognize that your body's worth isn't tied to its appearance but to its strength.

Negative thoughts will pop up. When our bodies change, it seems like it's all we can think about. When these pessimistic ideas arise, give them a quick, judgment-free acknowledgment, and then mentally reframe them. When you notice that you're focused on what you don't like about your body, take a moment to remind yourself of the incredible things your body has helped you achieve, like growing and nourishing a child.

As a woman, it's easy to get into the habit of constantly checking your appearance in every mirror you walk past or comparing your body to those of others around you. There were many times during my postpartum period when I felt a bit down about my body shape while looking in the mirror. This can be brutal for our self-image. Try to reduce the frequency of these behaviors by avoiding mirrors or simply using self-discipline. Or, go pick up your baby and look in the mirror again, to help cement the incredible truth of what your amazing body has accomplished in your mind. I did this many times during postpartum recovery, and it always improved my self-concept. Focus on how your body feels and functions, rather than how it looks on the outside.

Your body is smart; it knows what it needs to heal and recover. If it's sending you signals that it wants to rest, eat, or move, listen to and trust these signals by honoring your hunger, need for rest, or desire for activity when it arises. This probably isn't the best time to start CrossFit. You'll want to focus primarily on nourishing your body with foods and activities that make you feel good, promoting long-term health and well-being. Many women find it advantageous to stay in bed or on the couch for the first six weeks of the postpartum period. I did this for my second and third children, letting everyone come to me. Being able to let everything go for a moment to catch up on rest gave me the energy I needed to face the days ahead.

You are far more than a number on a scale or the size of your t-shirt. You're a mother, a partner, a friend, and so much more. Celebrate each of these facets regularly, and remind yourself of who you are beyond your physical appearance. If you reframe your thinking to focus on what your body has accomplished and take steps to support yourself holistically, you'll be well on your way to overcoming negative body image and embracing the new chapter of your life with confidence. After all, real beauty lies in self-love.

Our mind can be extremely powerful; if you're having a hard time embracing the changes in your body and reframing negative thoughts, consider using affirmations in your daily life to maintain a bit of control over your self-esteem. Affirmations can be repeated, either in your head or aloud, to support you in embracing your postpartum body. Here are a few you may want to incorporate into your routine:

- I am far more than what I look like.
- My body is strong, capable, and powerful.
- My body is a source of life and love.
- I nourish my body with love, respect, and care.
- I choose to love my body at every weight and every stage.
- I am patient and kind to myself as my body heals and adjusts.
- I release the pressure to "bounce back" to my pre-pregnancy body.
- I focus on what feels good to me.
- I listen to my body and honor its wishes.
- I celebrate my body for its strength and resilience.
- My body is amazing; look what it's achieved!
- I am grateful for my body's ability to heal, even if it takes time.
- The changes in my body are all a part of my personal motherhood story.
- Every change I observe is a reminder of the life I've created.
- My worth is not determined by any number.

Use these affirmations, or some of your own, to help cultivate a positive relationship with your body. The goal is to constantly remind yourself of the incredible strength and beauty you embody until you truly believe it.

Your body has quite literally brought new life into this world. Any changes that come as a result are just a testament to your resilience and adaptability. These changes should be approached with kindness and self-compassion to make this adjustment easier. Over time, you'll develop a more positive and accepting relationship with your body image.

Never hesitate to seek support from your family, friends, or professionals. You don't have to struggle alone—sharing your experiences can feel like a weight is lifted off your shoulders, and you might get some helpful encouragement as a result.

Going forward, continue to remind yourself of the remarkability of your body. You deserve to be proud of yourself at any stage in the process. The love and care you provide to your baby and yourself are far more important than fitting into your old jeans. Be gentle and patient with yourself, and engage in daily celebrations of the incredible feat you and your body have achieved together.

CHAPTER THREE

ESSENTIALS FOR NURTURERS TO FUEL THEIR POSTPARTUM RECOVERY

"Taking care of myself doesn't mean 'me first.' It means 'me too.'" [1]

L.R. KNOST

As mothers, our first instinct is often to put our babies' needs above our own. It seems like self-care isn't for us, but for whoever has the time to take long, luxurious baths and the money for pricey skincare products. Let me burst your bubble—self-care is absolutely essential for maintaining your well-being, and, therefore, the happiness of your family. To care for your child in the most nurturing way possible, you must first nourish yourself—and I mean literally. A happy, cared-for mama is just as well-fed as her child. Fueling your body with the right nutrients supports your recovery while sustaining your energy. After all, the fourth trimester isn't the end; it's just the beginning.

How you eat plays a massive role in your postpartum recovery, providing the nutrients you need to heal, regain strength, and support breastfeeding. Childbirth is a monumental task, and your body requires quite a bit of nourishment and a balanced diet to restore energy levels, repair tissues, and produce breast milk for your baby. Your diet should supply the necessary nutrients to support your body's healing processes and regulate your hormones. If you're breastfeeding, your body needs extra calories to provide quality milk. Let's take a look at what macronutrients a balanced meal includes:

- **Carbohydrates:** Your main source of energy, whole grains like oats, brown rice, and whole wheat bread provide sustained energy and are rich in fiber to aid in digestion.
- **Protein:** This macro aids in the repair of tissues and maintenance of muscle mass. Protein-rich foods like lean meats, poultry, fish, eggs, dairy products, beans, and legumes all support a healthy recovery process.
- **Healthy Fats:** Despite the universal fear related to the word "fat," this food group is actually necessary for effective hormone production and the maintenance of your brain health and overall energy. Include sources like avocados, nuts, seeds, and oily fish to make sure you're getting enough fatty acids.[2]

Still not sure what this means for your eating habits? The goal should be to have plenty of nutrient-dense foods with a variety of healing properties. Foods that are rich in protein and iron, like lean meats and poultry, are vital for rebuilding muscle tissue and replenishing any blood lost during birth. Oily fish are rich in omega-3 fatty acids, supporting your brain health and reducing inflammation. Foods that are high in vitamin C aid in tissue repair and support a productive immune system. Let's make a grocery list with some of the foods you should incorporate into your diet during the postpartum period:

- Chicken
- Eggs
- Turkey
- Black beans
- Pinto beans
- Salmon
- Mackerel
- Sardines
- Milk
- Yogurt
- Cheese
- Brown rice
- Quinoa
- Oats
- Oranges
- Lemons
- Strawberries
- Bell peppers[3]

In some traditions, like Traditional Chinese Medicine (TCM), it's believed that a mother's body can become too "cool" after childbirth. This prompts a need to consume warming, or "yang" foods during the postpartum period to restore a sense of balance. Aligning with this belief, foods like ginger, garlic, and warm soup are meant to stimulate circulation and promote healing. That being said, certain fruits and vegetables that are considered "cooling" (cucumbers, melons, etc.) should be consumed in moderation during this time.

This concept is specific to TCM, but the broader idea of finding balance in your diet during the postpartum period is universally important. Generally speaking, you should include a wide range of colors in your meals while focusing on antioxidants, vitamins, and minerals to support your healing.

I don't want you to start putting strict rules into your diet like "no cold foods" or "nothing that isn't immediately healing." Rather, you should be making mindful choices that nourish your body as much as you can, even if that means having a treat in between your meals. A balanced diet is chosen from a wide variety of food groups: vegetables, fruits, grains, proteins, and dairy. A healthy body needs a broad spectrum of nutrients to support recovery and milk production.

This one may seem obvious, but drinking plenty of water is significant to your breastfeeding experience. Try to keep a water bottle nearby at all times, or several that remain in various settings throughout your day. Sip on water throughout the day, not just when you feel the dry mouth coming on. Here's a tip: The giant cup with a bendy straw they often provide at the hospital is perfect for this, and similar styles can be found on Amazon or other online stores.

When you're nurturing a child, you may need to eat more than you're used to. According to the Centers for Disease Control and Prevention (CDC), a mother who's breastfeeding should consume anywhere from 2,300 to 2,500 calories a day, a bit more than non-breastfeeding women, who are suggested to consume 1,800 to 2,000 calories a day.[4] The extra nutrients may be difficult to make up for, but they are needed to support milk production and give you enough energy to care for your family.

If you're on a weight loss journey following your pregnancy, you might not want to hear that you're supposed to be eating more food than usual in your postpartum period. Your body, however, should be given the time and patience to recover at its own pace. This means approaching weight loss gradually rather than rushing yourself to get all the extra pounds off at once. Instead of starting new, hardcore exercise regimens and restricting your intake, focus on eating nutrient-dense foods that will keep you full for longer and engaging in gentle physical activity to strengthen your healing body.

Prenatal vitamins can help you get some of those essential nutrients you've been missing, even after childbirth. If you're struggling to achieve a balanced diet due to the demands of caring for a newborn, taking the same prenatal vitamins you had during your pregnancy, or introducing new ones into your routine, can fill in some of the nutritional gaps that arise after labor.

On a sleepless day, many of us want to reach for a cup of coffee (or five) to help us meet all the demands of new parenthood. I hate to be the bearer of bad news, but it's really best to limit caffeine in the fourth trimester. Caffeine can affect both your sleep and your baby's if you are breastfeeding. Similarly, alcohol should be consumed in moderation. Before nursing your child, make sure you've given your body enough time for the alcohol to clear from the breast milk.

Just like during your pregnancy, there are a few foods that should be avoided. While fish is a great source of omega-3s, certain fish, like shark, swordfish, and king mackerel are high in mercury and shouldn't be eaten while breastfeeding.

A balanced diet means avoiding foods that are high in sugar and unhealthy fats. This doesn't mean you should throw out every sweet treat you crave, but consuming sugary foods too often can contribute to energy crashes, while failing to provide the nutrients your body needs in the recovery process.

Getting enough sleep becomes a bit more of a challenge when you have a child, but it also becomes increasingly important during this time. Adequate sleep is necessary for emotional and physical healing, helping your body repair tissues, strengthen your immune system, and support your mental health. With a newborn, the idea of getting the rest you need may seem laughable. Many new mothers find themselves stuck in a cycle of exhaustion that can create a barrier to their healing process. The irregular sleep patterns of a young baby disrupts the sleep of everyone in the house, but the parents take the biggest hit. Add this to all of the stress that comes with caring for a new baby, worries about parenting, and shifts in your usual daily routine can make sleeping exceptionally difficult.

Many new mothers suffer from postpartum insomnia, a condition where they find it difficult to fall asleep, stay asleep, or return to sleep after waking up. A mother suffering from this will miss many opportunities to rest throughout the day, leaving them sleepless and running on empty. This condition can be particularly frustrating, as it often occurs in the midst of the overwhelming exhaustion that new parenthood brings.

Similar to regular insomnia, increased stressors, like the responsibilities and worries that come with caring for a newborn, can make it hard to relax enough for restful sleep. There's a near-constant need to respond to a baby's every need night and day, and these wakings can disrupt your sleep cycle and make it all the more difficult to get a full night's rest. After childbirth, there are also significant hormone fluctuations, which have an effect on your ability to sleep restfully. Conditions such as anxiety and depression also contribute to insomnia, and their symptoms are often triggered or worsened during the postpartum period.[5]

Sometimes it feels like struggles with postpartum insomnia never end, but its duration varies from person to person. It may resolve for some within a few weeks, as mothers adjust to their new routine and their baby begins to sleep more consistently. For others, insomnia can persist for much longer. If you feel like it's disrupted your life for a prolonged period of time, it might be time to reach out to a healthcare provider to explore relevant treatment options.

There are several routes you may take to improve your sleep quality. If the root of the issue lies in your child's inability to stay asleep, developing an understanding of your baby's sleep patterns can help you anticipate when you'll have chances to get some rest. As your baby gradually begins to sleep for longer periods, you will as well.

Restful sleep may be hidden behind tiny lifestyle modifications. Simple changes, like reducing caffeine intake and creating a calming bedtime environment, can make all the difference when it comes time to fall asleep. Many incorporate meditation or mindfulness into their nightly routine to induce relaxation and make it easier to drift away.

Going to bed and waking up at the same time each day can bring a drastic difference in your quality of sleep and make it easier to get restful sleep each night. Even if your nighttime sleep is interrupted, this routine will help you have a consistent mindset of R&R necessary for maintaining your energy levels.

To improve your quality of rest and your energy levels throughout the day, consider employing the following practical tips in your postpartum recovery routine:

1. **Sleep When the Baby Sleeps:** This strategy is simple, yet effective. Take advantage of every moment your baby catches up on rest, using it to do the same. Sometimes, this means letting go of other tasks for the time being.

2. **Schedule Regular Help:** Reach out to your partner, family, or friends to take over some of the baby care duties temporarily, allowing yourself to get a few hours of uninterrupted rest.

3. **Stay in "Rest Mode" When You Can't Sleep:** If you feel like you just can't fall asleep, try to stay in a restful state. Lie down, close your eyes, and practice deep breathing. Even if this doesn't prompt you to sleep, the rest you get can still be beneficial.

4. **Create a Partnered Nighttime Schedule:** If you're living with a partner or raising a child with a co-parent, consider creating a nighttime schedule that includes taking turns caring for the baby, so each of you gets a "shift" dedicated to resting.

5. **Follow Sleep Routines:** Establishing a consistent routine that includes meditation or making efforts to wind down can signal to your body that it's time to sleep and make the transition to rest easier.

6. **Find a Comfortable Position:** Sometimes rest is as easy as finding the right pose. After childbirth, it can be difficult to get cozy in a way that supports your comfort and recovery. The best postpartum sleep position tends to be on your back or side, as you can reduce any pressure

on your abdomen and pelvic area and allow for more restful sleep. If you've had a C-section, lying on your back with a pillow under your knees has been known to relieve pressure on the incision site. Figure out what works for you using pillows to support your body and make sleeping more comfortable.[6]

When it feels like a balanced diet and restful sleep aren't doing enough to support your physical and mental transition into motherhood, what you might be missing is exercise. Regular, gentle exercise after pregnancy offers a wide range of benefits for new mothers in the postpartum recovery phase. Pregnancy and childbirth place significant strain on your muscles, especially in the abdomen and pelvic floor. There are exercises designed to strengthen and tone the muscles to reduce the risk of complications, like diastasis recti and pelvic floor dysfunction, all while promoting a quicker recovery process.

If you gave birth vaginally, gentle exercise can help improve your recovery experience by improving circulation to speed up the healing process. Certain physical activities reduce discomfort by strengthening the muscles that support your pelvis and spine.

Even though it doesn't always feel like it immediately, regular exercise can boost your energy levels. New motherhood is often one of the most exhausting time periods in a person's life, and it can lead to depression and a general lack of energy. Exercise releases natural mood lifters (endorphins) that can help you feel more alert and less fatigued, even on your most sleepless nights.

It doesn't hurt that regular exercise contributes to weight loss. Many new mothers are eager to get back to their pre-pregnancy weight and strength. While strenuous activity is not recommended, a bit of regular, gentle practice combined with a balanced diet can help you get some of the excess weight off gradually and safely while improving your overall health and stamina.

It's not recommended to start exercises right away, though. Knowing when you're cleared to start a fitness regimen relies on a variety of factors, and it largely depends on the type of delivery you had and your overall health following childbirth. If you had a vaginal birth, you can usually get a recommendation to start gentle exercises like light walking or pelvic floor practices as soon as you feel ready.[7] Sometimes, this is even within the week you give birth. It's absolutely necessary to listen to your body and healthcare provider; rushing into intense activities is not recommended. Most healthcare professionals recommend waiting around six weeks before starting more vigorous exercises, like running, lifting, or climbing.

If you've had a cesarean section, it generally takes a bit longer to heal from childbirth than a vaginal birth. You need to spend extra time making sure your body has healed before starting any form of exercise, gentle or not. Most doctors recommend waiting at least six to eight weeks after a c-section before starting gentle exercises. Even then, you should always get clearance from your healthcare provider before starting a postpartum fitness routine to avoid recovery disruption.

Once you and your healthcare provider have agreed that you're ready to start exercising, there are a variety of low-risk activities that reintroduce movement and muscle growth to your routine and body. Here are a few gentle practices that you may benefit from once you're given the all-clear:

- **Abdominal Bracing:** Exercises that strengthen the core muscles that were stretched during pregnancy can be particularly beneficial for healing and preventing diastasis recti. Abdominal bracing involves tightening your ab muscles while sitting, standing, lying, or kneeling on all fours.

- **Pelvic Floor Exercises:** Often referred to as "kegels," pelvic floor exercises strengthen the muscles that support the bladder, uterus, and bowels. These can be started soon after either type of birth, and are helpful for preventing incontinence and supporting overall pelvic strength.

- **Walking:** An excellent low-impact exercise that can be started soon after childbirth, walking improves circulation, increases energy levels, and gradually helps to rebuild stamina without too much strain on your recovering body.

- **Swimming and Aqua Aerobics:** Once any postpartum bleeding has stopped and your incisions are healed, swimming and water-based aerobics are great ways to gently support your joints while providing a gentle, full-body workout.

- **Yoga and Pilates:** Exercises that improve your flexibility and strength, like yoga and Pilates, are great for rebuilding your core strength and enhancing your mental well-being. If needed, adjust an online or class-led yoga or Pilates routine to suit your postpartum body and help with stress relief during your recovery.

- **Low-Impact Aerobics:** Light dancing or elliptical machine usage can help gradually improve cardiovascular health and promote weight loss without the risk of injury or muscle strain.

- **Light Weight Training:** Intense weight lifting exercises are not recommended immediately after childbirth, but incorporating light weight training into your routine once you've had a chance to heal can help rebuild muscle strength and tone your body a bit. Start with small weights, like three or five pounds, and focus on consistent, controlled movements to avoid muscle strain.
- **Cycling:** Stationary cycling using a machine is a safe, low-impact option to improve your cardiovascular endurance and leg strength. If you're looking for a non-weight-bearing exercise to ease you back into fitness, cycling is a great choice.[8]

Returning to light exercise after pregnancy can feel very empowering, like taking a positive step toward reclaiming your strength and well-being. As a part of your recovery process, you'll want to make sure you're approaching any exercise routines with patience and listen to your body so that you're not rushing it into anything you're not physically ready for.

That being said, having enough energy to engage in effective exercise and get sufficient rest starts with a balanced diet. This may take a bit of time and adjusting to get right, but meal prepping for the week can make it a bit easier. Let's take a look at what a week of postpartum meal planning could look like:

Day 1

- **Breakfast:** Protein oatmeal
- **Snack:** Greek yogurt with honey and nuts
- **Lunch:** Korean seaweed soup (Miyeok Guk)
- **Snack:** Fresh fruit with almond/peanut butter

- **Dinner:** Autumn wild rice soup
- **Snack:** Chamomile latte

Day 2

- **Breakfast:** Rice congee
- **Snack:** Hard-boiled eggs with sea salt
- **Lunch:** Lemongrass, ginger, and lime chicken soup
- **Snack:** Sliced cucumber and hummus
- **Dinner:** Golden soup with pinto beans
- **Snack:** Spiced milk with ghee

Day 3

- **Breakfast:** Hot spiced milk with a slice of whole-grain toast
- **Snack:** Mixed berries
- **Lunch:** Kitchari
- **Snack:** Carrot sticks with guacamole
- **Dinner:** Immunity-boosting chicken soup

Day 4

- **Breakfast:** Protein oatmeal
- **Snack:** Walnuts and dried apricots
- **Lunch:** Sheng Hua Tang herbal soup
- **Snack:** Spinach, banana, and almond milk smoothie
- **Dinner:** Pepper soup
- **Snack:** Warm tea with milk and cinnamon

Day 5:

- **Breakfast:** Rice congee
- **Snack:** Sliced avocado with sea salt
- **Lunch:** Miyeok Guk
- **Snack:** Oatmeal cookies
- **Dinner:** Lemongrass, ginger, and lime chicken soup
- **Snack:** Chamomile latte

Of course, you don't have to follow the schedule you create to a T. If adjustments need to be made to support your caloric intake or energy levels, be sure to do so. Sometimes, you just get a craving! Don't put off these feelings; try treating them with similar, healthy alternatives, or simply allow yourself a moment of indulgence every once and a while.

If you're looking for a bit of inspiration, try some of the following postpartum recipes that are used in different cultures throughout the world:

Kitchari (Ayurvedic Bean Dish)

Ingredients:

- 1/2 cup split yellow mung dal (lentils)
- 1/2 cup basmati rice
- 6 cups water
- 1 tbsp ghee or butter
- 1 tsp cumin seeds
- 1 tsp mustard seeds
- 1 tsp turmeric powder
- 1/2 tsp ground coriander
- 1/2 tsp ground fennel

- 1/2 tsp ground ginger
- 1/4 tsp hing (asafoetida)
- 1 small carrot, chopped
- 1 small zucchini, chopped
- Fresh cilantro for garnish
- Salt to taste

Instructions:

1. Rinse the mung dal and rice under cold water.
2. In a large pot, heat the ghee or butter over medium heat. Add cumin and mustard seeds and heat until aromatic.
3. Add turmeric, coriander, fennel, ginger, and hing. Stir to combine.
4. Add the mung dal and rice, coating it with the spices.
5. Pour in water and bring it to a boil. Reduce heat, cover, and simmer for 25-30 minutes, until the grains are soft.
6. Add chopped veggies and cook for another 10 minutes, until tender.
7. Season and garnish with fresh cilantro.

Hot Spiced Milk with Ghee

Ingredients:

- 1 cup organic whole milk or non-dairy alternative
- 1 tsp ghee
- 1/4 tsp turmeric
- 1/4 tsp ground ginger
- 1/4 tsp cinnamon
- A pinch of black pepper
- Honey or maple syrup to taste

Instructions:

1. Heat the milk in a small saucepan over medium heat. Get it warm, but avoid boiling.
2. Stir in the ghee or butter, turmeric, ginger, cinnamon, and black pepper.
3. Heat for another minute, stirring constantly.
4. Remove from heat and sweeten with honey or maple syrup.
5. Serve warm.

Simple and Cozy Autumn Wild Rice Soup

Ingredients:

- 1 cup wild rice, rinsed
- 2 tbsp olive oil
- 1 onion, diced
- 2 carrots, diced
- 2 celery stalks, diced
- 3 garlic cloves, minced
- 6 cups vegetable or chicken broth
- 1 tsp dried thyme
- 1/2 tsp ground sage
- Salt and pepper to taste
- 1/2 cup heavy cream or coconut milk (optional)
- Fresh parsley for garnish

Instructions:

1. In a large pot, heat the olive oil over medium heat. Add the onion, carrots, celery, and garlic, and sauté until softened.
2. Add the wild rice, broth, thyme, sage, salt, and pepper. Bring to a boil, then reduce heat and simmer for 45-50 minutes until the rice is tender.
3. Stir in the cream or coconut milk if using, and heat through.
4. Garnish with fresh parsley before serving.

Immunity Boosting Chicken Soup

Ingredients:

- 1 whole chicken, cut into pieces
- 1 tbsp olive oil
- 1 onion, diced
- 3 garlic cloves, minced
- 2 carrots, sliced
- 2 celery stalks, sliced
- 1 sweet potato, diced
- 1 tsp turmeric
- 1 tsp ground cumin
- 8 cups chicken broth
- Salt and pepper to taste
- Fresh cilantro for garnish

Instructions:

1. Heat olive oil over medium heat in a large pot. Add onion and garlic and heat until fragrant.
2. Add chicken pieces and cook until browned on all sides.
3. Stir in veggies, turmeric, and cumin. Cook for 5 minutes.
4. Pour in chicken broth and bring the mixture to a boil. Reduce heat to a simmer for 45 minutes.
5. Remove the chicken pieces, shred the meat, and return it to the pot.
6. Season and garnish with fresh cilantro.

Chamomile Latte

Ingredients:

- 1 cup whole milk or dairy-free alternative
- 1 chamomile tea bag
- 1 tbsp honey
- ¼ tsp ground cinnamon

Instructions:

1. Heat the milk in a small saucepan until warm.
2. Remove from heat and add the tea bag. Steep for 5 minutes.
3. Remove the bag, stir in honey, and sprinkle with cinnamon.
4. Serve warm.

Rice Congee

Ingredients:

- 1 cup jasmine rice
- 8 cups water or broth
- 1 inch ginger, sliced
- 2 cloves garlic, minced
- Salt to taste
- Green onions and soy sauce

Instructions:

1. Rinse the rice under cold water.
2. Bring water or broth to a boil in a large pot. Add the rice, ginger, and garlic.
3. Reduce heat and simmer for 1 to 1.5 hours, stirring occasionally until the rice breaks down and the mixture reaches a porridge-like texture.
4. Season and garnish with green onions and soy sauce.
5. Serve warm.

These recipes can be a starting point for your personalized meal-prepping schedule. Each one is hand-picked from a variety of cultures and traditions in order to support the functioning of a postpartum body, providing you with the right balance of whole grains and proteins to aid your recovery process.

By now, you get it: proper nutrition and self-care are vital components of your postpartum recovery. Your body deserves and needs wholesome foods and gentle exercises to support the physical and emotional healing that occurs after childbirth. It's not a luxury to take care of yourself and nourish your body—it's a necessity. It allows you to be the best and happiest mother you can be.

We'll next address the emotional and mental challenges that come with the postpartum period. It's normal to struggle during this time, but a variety of methods can be used to guide your motherhood voyage and make the process a bit easier. We'll look into time-honored approaches that offer additional support and help you create a well-rounded, tailored care plan.

NAVIGATING BABY BLUES AND POSTPARTUM DEPRESSION

"Bad moments don't make bad mamas." [1]

LYSA TERKEURST

Three months after the birth of my second child, I was sobbing on the phone as I poured my heart out to a woman whom I believed to be a therapist. After informing me that she was only the appointment coordinator for the psychiatry department, she told me that many of their mental health specialists were on strike that summer, but that she could get me an appointment with a therapist in three months. I thanked her and hung up, feeling more isolated and lost than I had before. It was the beginning of the Covid-19 pandemic in 2020, and I'd been struggling with practically every aspect of my life, feeling too ashamed of my negative feelings to share them with anyone. Transitioning from one to two children had not been easy for our family, and I was working from our remote, rural home without childcare. Just like many other moms who struggled with mental health issues after pregnancy, I didn't know where to turn. This chapter will outline some of the insight I gained as I learned to manage my symptoms.

Even in your most challenging, emotional moments, your worth as a mother remains intact. The postpartum period is likely filled with one of the widest ranges of emotions you've been through. New mothers experience joy, love, and fulfillment to the furthest extent, all while battling persistent feelings of anxiety, sadness, and doubt. Sometimes, these feelings get so intense that it's easy to lose sight of the truth. Even when you're struggling, these negative perceptions are not a reflection of your ability to care for your child or be a valuable mother; they are part of the natural process that occurs when you're adjusting to the changes that come with bringing new life into the world. Navigating these emotions is not always easy, but it seems a lot more possible when you understand why you feel the way you do.

The hormonal changes that occur after giving birth are . . . plentiful. Significant shifts in your body occur during the recovery from pregnancy and childbirth, and these can have an intense impact on your emotional well-being during this time. In the first few weeks after giving birth, your body starts to experience a dramatic drop in the levels of progesterone and estrogen.[2] These hormones play crucial roles in maintaining your pregnancy, and their sudden drop can lead to mood swings, feelings of sadness and irritability, and physical changes like hair loss or skin dryness. These fluctuations are commonly referred to as the "baby blues," a lighthearted way of describing the emotional impact that a body's changes have on a new mother.

When you're pregnant, the progesterone in your body has a calming effect. When this hormone drops, you can feel anxious, irritable, and downright sad. Similarly, a drop in estrogen levels is usually the culprit behind a new mother's intense mood swings, as well as other physical symptoms like night sweats and vaginal dryness. Your Oxytocin levels also take a big hit. Often referred to as the "love hormone," oxytocin helps you bond with your baby and promote feelings of attachment, as well as supporting milk ejection during nursing. When this hormone fluctuates, as it often does, it can have detrimental effects on your emotional stability, causing ups and downs and feelings of stress that occur when breastfeeding challenges arise. Lastly, prolactin, the hormone responsible for milk production, tends to increase after childbirth. While it's supposed to help you with the production of breastmilk, high levels of prolactin can cause you to feel fatigued and it can even suppress ovulation, delaying the stability of your menstrual cycle.[3]

By the time you reach the three-month mark after giving birth, your hormones are starting to stabilize, but they're not quite back in their pre-pregnancy groove. Many women start to see their menstrual cycle returning at this point, which is more likely to occur when you're not breastfeeding. For mothers who are nursing, prolactin often remains elevated and has an impact on their mood and energy. Progesterone and estrogen gradually start to normalize after three months. You may notice an improvement in your mood swings or other emotional instability, but it varies from mother to mother.

These hormonal changes are not insignificant. They affect nearly everything, from your daily mood and energy levels to your overall physical health, and their fluctuations are often the reason behind the baby blues, postpartum depression, and symptoms like fatigue, headaches, and appetite changes.

Just like the rest of your body, hormones don't immediately go back to normal in the fourth trimester. It can take up to a year or more for some women to reach normal hormonal levels, depending on factors like breastfeeding, stress levels, and overall health. Everyone's experience is different, and there's really no one-size-fits-all answer when it comes to hormonal stabilization.

While you can't avoid the effects that hormonal fluctuation has on your body and mind, there are a few strategies you can incorporate into your daily life to mitigate their impact. For example, hormonal changes often lead to heightened cravings for sugary foods, but giving in to these cravings each time can cause spikes and blood sugar crashes. This can worsen your mood swings and fatigue. Instead, try focusing on balanced meals that provide enough protein, healthy fats, and complex carbohydrates to keep you satiated, and enough yumminess to curb those cravings.

Sleep is another crucial aspect of balanced hormonal levels. Getting enough rest can be challenging, but using the advice from Chapter Three can ease some of this difficulty. Try to nap when your baby naps, and never hesitate to ask a partner, family member, or friend for a bit of help.

Regular physical activity boosts your endorphins, which are natural mood lifters that can help to counteract the effects of hormonal fluctuations. Try using some of the gentle activities from the last chapter, like walking, yoga, or pilates, to help you feel more energized and less *blegh*.

Hormonal changes can be challenging, but they're a natural part of the postpartum experience. Be patient with yourself, and remember that these changes are temporary. With time, your body will adjust to a new normal, especially with the help of dietary improvements, restful sleep, and exercise.

The baby blues might sound like no big deal, but they can cause some serious disruptions to a mother's life. This temporary condition is categorized as feelings of sadness, anxiety, and mood swings that arise after the birth of a new child. Around 80 percent of us experience the baby blues after birth (that's four out of five!)[4] It's not exactly ideal to feel like you're going through an emotional rollercoaster when you're supposed to be focused on raising a new child, but the good news is that you're not alone. Chances are, a new mama around you is going through something similar.

The baby blues have a tendency to pop up a few days after giving birth, and they can last up to a month. During this time, many new mothers find themselves experiencing a range of emotional symptoms. Let's take a look:

- **Crying Inexplicably:** It's not uncommon for new mothers to feel "weepy" or randomly burst into tears over seemingly minor triggers, or for no apparent reason at all.
- **Mood Swings:** You may feel like your emotions swing from happiness to hopelessness at the drop of a dime, or that you feel particularly irritable and sensitive.
- **Feeling Unattached:** Some mothers feel a lack of connection with their newborn in the first couple of weeks. This can be incredibly distressing, especially with the pressure to bond with a new baby, but it's totally normal.
- **Missing Your Old Life:** You might long for the freedom you once had to go out with friends or act irresponsibly. Many mothers miss aspects of their lives before they had a child, especially in the first month postpartum.

- **Feeling Anxious About Your Baby:** It's common to have heightened, overwhelming concerns about your baby's well-being. Even when there's no specific cause for worry, many new mothers are ridden with anxiety about their baby's safety or health.
- **Restlessness and Insomnia:** Even the most exhausted mothers sometimes struggle to fall asleep or stay asleep. This can lead to further exhaustion, elevating your negative feelings throughout the day.
- **Brain Fog and Indecisiveness:** Simple tasks can feel a lot more overwhelming when you're in your baby blues. You might struggle with concentration or decision-making.[5]

The good news about the baby blues is that they usually only last a few days to a few weeks. This short-lived period coincides with the time your hormone levels are fluctuating rapidly, and they can feel intense at first. Regardless, they typically resolve on their own, as your body and mind start to adjust to the new demands of motherhood. When you're in the depths of it, though, you can make a couple of changes to your regimen to make sure you're not getting caught up in those negative feelings.

As with any mental or physical challenge, getting as much sleep as possible can help you recover from the baby blues more quickly. Nourishing your body with healthy foods and getting outside for some fresh air and sunlight can make you feel better physically, which often prompts a happier mindset. Don't be afraid to suffer on your own; Reach out to a partner, a family member, or a friend to talk about what you're going through and find a bit of emotional support. It's also not selfish to take a few moments every day to do something that brings you joy, like reading a book, listening to a podcast, or making yourself a fancy meal to wind down at the end of the day.

With all the stress in your life, it can be easy to neglect the relationship you have with your spouse or partner. This can add tension to the relationship, and it doesn't usually help with the baby blues. Taking extra steps to strengthen your bond with your partner can give you a bit of emotional support while helping both of you feel less isolated. You're both experiencing a newborn together, so be sure to share insights as you go, talk about your feelings, and make an effort to spend time together.

When you're going through emotional turbulence after pregnancy, it's important to look out for more serious, persistent symptoms that sometimes seem like they might be the baby blues, but are actually signs of a serious mental health condition. Postpartum depression (PPD) is more intense than the short-lived baby blues, and it lasts longer, significantly impacting a mother's ability to care for herself and her baby. PPD is serious, and it's not just a sign of weakness or a bad mood that someone can "snap out of." It requires special attention, care, and sometimes professional intervention to overcome.[6]

The baby blues (BBs) and PPD share a few similarities, but the BBs are typically a lot less serious than the ladder. Postpartum depression, on the other hand, can begin anytime within the first year of motherhood and tends to last for a prolonged period of time. PPD is also much less common, affecting only about 10-20 percent of mothers. Here's what it can look like:

- **Trouble Sleeping:** Mothers with PPD experience difficulty falling or staying asleep, even when they're exhausted.

- **Appetite Disruptions:** Significant changes in your appetite, like eating too much or less than usual, may be indicative of postpartum depression.
- **Severe Fatigue:** PPD often comes with extreme tiredness that doesn't seem to improve with rest.
- **Lowered Libido:** Women experiencing postpartum depression often go through a noticeable decrease in sexual drive or desire.
- **Frequent Mood Changes:** Rapid mood swings, from deep sadness to irritability and anger, are common PPD symptoms.
- **Disinterest in your Child:** Some mothers who are suffering from PPD will feel completely disconnected from their baby for a prolonged period.
- **Frequent Crying:** Frequent, uncontrollable crying without a clear reason, can be a sign of postpartum depression.
- **Depressed Mood:** A persistent feeling of sadness and emptiness is the central emotion for those who are suffering from this condition.
- **Severe Anger:** Feeling uncharacteristically angry or irritable may be a sign of PPD.
- **Loss of Pleasure:** A symptom known as anhedonia may prompt a loss of interest in activities you once enjoyed.
- **Feelings of Worthlessness and Hopelessness:** Negative thoughts are plentiful when you suffer from PPD, and they can impede your confidence in your ability to care for yourself or your baby.
- **Trouble Concentrating:** Difficulty focusing or remembering things is a common PPD symptom.

- **Thoughts of Death:** In severe cases, a suffering mother may have thoughts of self-harm or suicide, signaling the need for immediate professional intervention.
- **Thoughts of Violence:** Postpartum depression can prompt intrusive thoughts about harming a newborn or someone else, which is a severe mental emergency.[7]

Postpartum depression can get very real, very quickly. If you feel like you align with some of the symptoms of PPD, it's probably a sign to give yourself and your mind some extra attention and care, and even sometimes pursue immediate medical care.

While the exact source of postpartum depression is not fully understood, there are a variety of physical, emotional, and environmental factors that are believed to contribute to this condition. Let's take a look at some of these:

- **Mental Health History:** Many women with a history of depression or premenstrual dysphoric disorder, like those who have suffered from it before or during their pregnancy, are at a higher risk for PPD than others. Familial history makes a difference, too. Mothers with depression, bipolar disorder, or other mood-altering conditions in their family tree can have an increased risk.
- **Age:** Surprisingly, younger mothers, particularly those in their teens or early twenties, are more likely to develop this condition.
- **Mood About Pregnancy:** Mixed or negative feelings about a pregnancy are contributing factors, increasing the risk of developing depression after childbirth.

- **Stress:** Significant stressors like the loss of a job or the death of a loved one, if aligned with your pregnancy and fourth trimester, can prompt symptoms of PPD. Even just the stress of caring for a newborn and concerns about your parenting abilities can lead to anxiety, which is a substantial trigger for postpartum depression.
- **Health of Newborn:** Having a baby who requires special needs or has health problems can have an impact on a mother's mental state.
- **Isolation:** Single mothers or those who live far from family and friends are more likely to suffer from postpartum depression. A lack of a strong support network can leave new mothers feeling overwhelmed and helpless. Strained relationships with a partner can also contribute to the development of PPD.
- **Hormonal Imbalance:** The sharp drop in thyroid hormones, or others such as estrogen and progesterone, can trigger mood swings and lead to fatigue and depression.
- **Lack of Sleep:** Chronic sleep deprivation is common in new mothers, but it can elevate feelings of fatigue, irritability, and depression.
- **Low Self-Image:** Many mothers struggle with changes in their body and identity after birth, which can prompt feelings of inadequacy and postpartum depression.

Postpartum depression, if left untreated, can lead to serious complications. It can mean the start of chronic depression, affecting your long-term health and creating a permanent issue. It can interfere with your relationship with your child in various ways, making bonding more difficult and impacting your child's emotional development negatively. These problems can branch out into the relationships you have with your partner, family members, and friends, further isolating you and increasing the amount of conflict and stress in your life.

In severe cases, postpartum depression can lead to thoughts of suicide. If this occurs, immediate and professional intervention is necessary.

Even if you're not struggling with thoughts of self-harm, there is never shame in seeking professional help to aid in the recovery process and prevent further complications. Treatment for PPD can look like many things, and it often includes a combination of therapy, medication, and daily activities related to nurturing your mental health. Many women who struggle find that with the right support, they are able to make a full recovery that allows them to enjoy their time with their newborn.

Knowing when to seek professional help is your superpower. If your symptoms persist for more than two weeks, you feel unable to care for yourself or your baby, you experience thoughts of harming yourself or others, or your symptoms seem to worsen over time, it's time to make that call. In a scenario where you're unable to seek professional care and there's no immediate threat to your safety, try to do everything you can (reaching out to others for support, taking time off work, etc.) to support your mental health and reach a position where you're able to enjoy the relationship between you and your newborn. Seeking help is the first step toward feeling better. With the right treatment, postpartum depression is highly treatable, and you may completely regain and enhance your well-being and confidence.

We've touched on mindfulness and its ability to support your mental health, but let's really get into what this powerful concept is capable of. Mindfulness is the practice of being present and engaged in the current moment without any adjustment to your thoughts, feelings, and surroundings. Being mindful means paying attention to everything going on inside and around you, rather than staying lost in thoughts about the past or concerns about the future.[8] Many moms choose to support their mental and physical recovery by using mindful techniques like meditation and breathing exercises, or by focusing on daily activities with a sense of consciousness.

Mindfulness innately encourages you to treat yourself with the same kindness and understanding you extend to your friends. In the postpartum period, this self-compassion is particularly important. If you're focused on the present moment, you're less likely to ruminate on fears about the future, which can hold you back and leave you feeling overwhelmed by the responsibilities of new motherhood. Embracing the here and now offers you a fresh perspective, one where you can actually appreciate each and every little moment with your baby, even the hard ones. While many mothers miss out on fleeting moments of joy in parenthood, mindfulness keeps others fully present and able to enjoy each memory created with her family.

Practicing mindfulness has its effects on the body, too. While many mothers battle sleep deprivation, being mindful helps others navigate their exhaustion and learn to rest their bodies as much as possible. It can also support emotional regulation, helping you observe your emotions without any judgment and process them in a healthy way. A lot of people make realizations during theory mindfulness practices that help them be more honest about their needs, making it easier to recognize when they need to ask for help or support from others.

The beauty of being mindful is in its simplicity. In fact, just a few quick changes in your daily routine can make you a more mindful, present person and mother. For example, a daily morning routine that supports mindfulness might follow a schedule like this one:

1. Wake up gently, spending the first few moments of consciousness stretching and taking deep breaths.
2. Engage in mindful breathing by sitting quietly for 5 minutes and focusing on your breathing. Inhale slowly, hold for a few seconds, and then exhale completely.
3. Use a gratitude practice: think of three things you're grateful for upon waking up, like a good night's rest or the gentle sound of your baby's breaths.
4. Set an intention for the day, reflecting on how you want to approach the time you have. Consider setting an intention of patience, joy, or self-compassion.

Being mindful once isn't enough, and consistency is required for results. Check in with yourself daily by taking a moment out of your routine to ask yourself how you're feeling, what you need, and whether you're being kind to yourself. This quick checklist connects you to your well-being and keeps you in the know so you can make adjustments to your mindset if you have to.

When responsibilities start to pile up and you're just downright overwhelmed, mindfulness is there to keep it simple. Take a deep breath and be present in the moment, asking yourself what single priority you should focus on rather than trying to take it all at once. This practice can reduce your stress and make it easier to manage the challenges you're facing throughout the day.

If you're looking to incorporate some mindfulness into your day, the ABCDEFG meditation is a great starting point. It's designed to help moms center themselves and find a bit of calm amidst the daily chaos. Here's how to practice ABCDEFG meditation:[9]

- **Awareness:** The first step is to become completely aware of your current state, acknowledging the physical, mental, and emotional feelings you're experiencing. Take a moment to notice how you feel without judging it or trying to change it.
- **Breathe:** Take a deep breath through your nose, filling your lungs. Hold for a moment, and then exhale the air slowly through your mouth. Repeat this while focusing on the sensation of the breath entering and leaving your lungs.
- **Center:** As you breathe, bring your attention to the center of your body, right below your rib cage. Imagine this area as your center of gravity, a calm, warm light emanating from it as it grounds you and brings you stability.
- **Drop:** Drop your shoulders and release any tension in your body by unclenching your hands and feet or loosening your tightened muscles. Imagine yourself letting go of any stress or worries you're holding onto, melting them away with each exhale.
- **Expand:** Expand your awareness out from your center and take note of the space around you. Feel the ground beneath your feet and the air on your skin, feeling supported by your surroundings.
- **Focus:** Choose a word or phrase that brings you peace, like "calm," "relax," or "I am enough." Silently repeat this word or phrase to yourself with each inhale and let it anchor you in the present moment.

- **Gratitude:** End the meditation with a reflection. Jot down a few things you are grateful for following your session, like a cozy house or the love you hold for your child. Take a moment to imagine this gratitude filling your heart and body.

This practice is mostly conducted internally, so it can be taken with you anywhere and at any time. Your feelings of overwhelm or negativity can be reduced within as little as five minutes, making it a perfect practice for moms who often only have that much time to take out of their day anyway.

Postnatal yoga offers numerous benefits for new mothers to support their physical and emotional health simultaneously. Yoga aids in the physical and mental recovery that occurs after childbirth. It strengthens core muscles, like the abdomen and pelvic floor, prompting improved posture and reducing back pain. It gradually builds your flexibility to make general mobility easier, especially beneficial as your body is adjusting to so many changes after birth. Yoga also incorporates mindfulness and breathing exercises to reduce stress and promote a sense of relaxation, which literally *every* mother could benefit from. Here's a routine that you can incorporate into your life to gently and gradually strengthen your body while promoting calmness:

Plank Vinyasa

1. Start in a tabletop position on your hands and knees.
2. Step your feet back and come into a plank position, with your body in a straight line from head to heels.
3. Hold the plank, keep your hips level, and take a deep breath to engage your core.

4. Lower your knees to the floor, then lower your chest and chin, keeping your elbows close to your body.

5. Push through your hands, lifting your chest into a gentle cobra pose. Stretch your back and open your chest.

6. Exhale and push into a child's pose while sitting on your heels and extending your arms forward.

7. Moving with your breathing patterns, repeat this flow 3-5 times.

Locust Post (Salabhasana)

1. Lie face down on your mat or rug with your arms by your sides and your palms facing down.

2. Take a deep breath and use the inhale to lift your head, chest, and legs off the ground at once.

3. Engage your back muscles, keeping your gaze slightly forward and your neck long.

4. Hold this pose for 3-5 breaths and gently lower it back down.

5. Repeat this flow 2-3 times.

Pelvic Tilts

1. Lie on your back, knees bent and feet flat and hip-width apart.

2. Keep your arms by your sides, palms facing down.

3. Inhale and tilt your pelvis upward while flattening your lower back against the floor.

4. Exhale, tilting your pelvis downward and arching your lower back away from the floor.

5. Continue this rocking motion while moving with your breath from 10-15 repetitions.

Legs Wide Pose (Upavistha Konasana)

1. Sit on the floor with your legs extended out to the sides.
2. Flex your feet, engage your thigh muscles, and place your hands on the floor in front of you.
3. Gentle walk your hands forward, hinging at your hips.
4. Keep your spine long and avoid rounding your back. Hold the stretch for 5-150 breaths, feeling a gentle pull in your thighs and hamstrings.

Scissors

1. Lie on your back, arms by your sides and legs extended straight up toward the ceiling.
2. Engage your core and slowly lower your right leg toward the floor. Keep your left leg extended upward.
3. Inhale and switch sides, bringing your right leg up and lowering the left one.
4. Continue alternating legs in a controlled motion for 10-12 repetitions.[10]

After childbirth, the path toward rebuilding strength and flexibility should be a gradual one. Listen to your body as you go and don't push yourself too hard, especially if you're recovering from a complicated childbirth or a cesarean section. Gentle practices like postnatal yoga can be powerful aids in your physical recovery, helping your emotional well-being in the process.

The postpartum period is a time of immense change, so it naturally brings about quite some turbulence in your emotional regulation. As long as you continue to support your own healing, understand the difference between the baby blues and postpartum depression, and recognize when you need to seek professional help, you'll be well on your way to supporting yourself and your family.

Incorporating mindfulness into your routine can be an added layer of support, helping you manage stress, stay present, and promote a greater sense of self-compassion that's needed for a successful fourth trimester. In the following chapter, we'll look even deeper into the self-care practices that are designed specifically for new moms to nurture and help them navigate the early stages of motherhood.

CHAPTER FIVE

SELF-CARE PRACTICES FOR POSTPARTUM MOMS

"Just because I can do it all doesn't mean I have to do it all." [1]

G. MICHELLE GOODLOE

When I was a new mother, I felt the weight of society's pressure pushing down on my shoulders. It seemed like most moms were somehow able to "do it all," even at the expense of their own well-being. While we're sometimes capable of managing so many responsibilities at once, it doesn't mean we should. Making time for self-care is the only way to maintain your health and sanity and become the best mother you can be. There's a reason you're instructed to put on your own oxygen mask before helping others on a plane; you can't take care of others if you haven't taken care of your own needs first.

Practicing postpartum self-care means making intentional steps to tend to your physical, emotional, and mental needs following the birth of a child. Let's be real, mamas don't usually have all of the time in the world to pamper themselves. That being said, it's even more important for mothers to allow themselves time to replenish their energy, heal from the physical strain that comes with childbirth, and acknowledge the emotions they're feeling.

Early parenting can take a significant toll on mothers who feel societal or internal pressure to constantly prioritize their baby's needs over their own. For some reason, postpartum self-care is not always the most popular topic. In reality, it's a crucial part of being a good mom. The more you care for yourself, the better the position you're in to care for your baby. There's nothing selfish about working to regain your strength and stabilize your emotions, and these efforts all help you be a more present mother for your child.[2]

I get it—it's not always easy to find time to care for yourself in a busy postpartum schedule. You're going to have to move your routine around little by little until it becomes a natural part of your day. Here are a few examples:

- You wake up a few minutes early to enjoy a cup of tea in the morning while the baby is still asleep. Normally, you'd be rushing to get out of bed after waking up to the sound of crying.
- You ask someone else to help lift a few heavy objects around the house to protect your body as it's healing.
- You schedule and attend multiple postpartum doctor appointments to check in with your body and mind. You are sure to review your concerns with the professional.
- You say "yes" to help from friends and family. You allow them to do some of your chores and baby care.
- You say "no" without guilt to visitors when you're overwhelmed.

- You set aside time throughout the day to do something you enjoy, like reading, meditating, or listening to music, even if it's brief.
- When you're completing tasks or caring for the baby, incorporate activities you love as much as possible by playing your favorite playlist, audiobook, or podcast to multitask.
- Take your baby on walks to get a bit of physical exercise and fresh air—walks are natural mood boosters.
- When you have the time, give yourself an at-home beauty treatment using face masks or manicure materials to feel rejuvenated after a long day or tough morning.
- Write self-care tasks into your schedule so you're more likely to stick to your regimen.

With a bit of planning, these simple practices can fit into even the busiest days and bring you closer to your postpartum recovery goals. Setting boundaries is another part of self-care that is often understated or ignored, but doing so is a communicative way to protect your space and mindset. The postpartum period can be an especially vulnerable time for new mothers who are trying to adjust to new emotional and physical demands. You may notice, during this time, that nearly everyone wants to offer advice, visit you and the baby, or help out (even when it doesn't really align with what you need). While your friends and family are usually well-intentioned, sometimes all of this can be overwhelming and it might take away from your personal recovery and the relationship you're building with your baby.

Communicating your needs and boundaries sometimes seems scary, but it's a healthy way to create an environment that serves to protect you and your family. Mental exhaustion is a common feeling among new mothers, and they often feel like they just have to keep going. Luckily, this isn't the case. Boundaries can prevent burnout from constantly saying "yes," and avoid the unnecessary stress that comes with it. During your fourth trimester, you should have two priorities: to tend to the well-being of you and your family and to build a relationship with your child. To do this, you'll need to control the flow of visitors by sometimes saying "no," and to be honest, you'll probably have to ignore some of the advice you're given, too. Moms often feel like they should be overextended, even when it takes a significant toll on their own happiness.[3] It's not always easy to figure out exactly what you need to do to protect your space. Here are some of the boundaries you may want to consider incorporating into your relationships during the postpartum period:

1. Limit visitation during the early days to give yourself more time to recover and adjust to the schedule you and your baby are on.
2. Let others know when they'd be welcome, and when you'd need some family time.
3. Decide how long visitors can stay, depending on your energy and stress levels. Keep visits short if you're not feeling up for it.
4. If others caring for your baby makes you uncomfortable, specify which types of tasks you'd like to get help from, like laundry, cooking, or running errands.
5. Politely but firmly let others know when their advice isn't needed, especially when the values of the advice don't align with your own.
6. When friends or family seem to get a bit *too* invested, limit what information you share and communicate only what you're comfortable sharing. Mothers often feel

obligated to share every detail about their postpartum or baby care experiences.

7. Choose who you allow into your support circle based on how their actions align with your needs. Not everyone is a positive influence and you and your family are more vulnerable to negative advice or energy during your postpartum period.

The hardest part of setting healthy boundaries is determining exactly what your needs are. Once you've done that, your role is to discuss them with your friends and family, outlining your expectations and preferences. Many of us have been taught that setting boundaries makes us mean or cold, but the guilt that follows this mindset is completely unnecessary and unhelpful. Healthy boundaries exist to benefit you and your family, and there's nothing selfish about saying no sometimes. You're not ungrateful or rude, you're simply acknowledging your own well-being. If you're anything like me, setting boundaries is not the easiest thing in the world. If you're anticipating a bit of difficulty with these conversations, practice role-playing with a partner or friend to feel more confident. That being said, there may still be instances where you have to adjust your boundaries slightly for the well-being of your family.

Self-compassion is a major component in your emotional healing process. As defined by psychologist Dr. Kristin Neff, self-compassion is the act of treating yourself with the same kindness and understanding that you would offer to a friend in difficult times.[4] Similarly, self-love is the practice of accepting yourself fully as you are and taking time to care for your own well-being. Both of these concepts involve making choices that nourish and support your body while approaching yourself with empathy. During a time so full of emotional highs and lows, self-love and compassion are a must.

Self-criticism is normal, and it can become heightened during the fourth trimester. Whether you're a new parent or doing it all over again, you're exploring a world that may be unfamiliar or overwhelming. The constant struggle with baby care and second-guessing yourself combined with the pressure of having a human's development in your hands can lead to feelings of inadequacy. Self-compassion serves as a reminder that perfection is not required, and struggling is a part of the process. Practicing love and care for yourself is required to develop resilience and emotional balance during one of the most transformative periods in your life.

Here are a few ways to encourage a sense of self-love and compassion during early parenthood:

- Remain absolutely present in the moment, observing your thoughts and emotions judgment-free. When things feel too much, ground yourself in what's in front of you.
- Treat yourself with care and kindness similar to the way you treat your beloved friends. When self-criticism makes its way in, challenge it with gentle thoughts.
- Seek support from people who understand your journey: friends, family, or support groups.
- Even if it's only 10 minutes, take a break throughout the day to engage in self-care practices.
- Embrace each part of the process, even the imperfect ones. Motherhood is messy and unpredictable—even the best mother makes mistakes; she just learns from them.
- Motherhood changes you and your priorities, but it shouldn't take away who you were before. Dedicate time

to yourself to rediscover passions, hobbies, and pieces of your identity you aligned with before motherhood.

- Take care of yourself when you're stressed to avoid burnout or more intense emotional releases. When you feel anxiety creeping up, place your hand over your head, take deep breaths, and name a few things you're grateful for in the present moment.

- You're not going to get everything the first time, and you don't have to. Be patient with yourself and gentle as you navigate the complicated aspects of being a parent.

- Make choices that consistently align with your priorities and values; staying true to yourself is a form of self-love in itself.[5]

One of the biggest culprits behind unnecessary stress and emotional challenges that new mothers suffer from is the unrealistic expectations set upon them. Depending on your current circumstances, resources, and abilities, you won't be able to achieve it all, and that's okay! When you're setting goals, it can be tempting to make them as large-scale as possible, but being realistic about what you'll be able to achieve means that you won't have to deal with the unnecessary disappointment that comes with trying to reach impractical objectives. The postpartum period is riddled with overwhelming emotions, stress, and exhaustion that can often make productivity more difficult.[6] That's okay; adjusting to motherhood is not easy, and it's important to give yourself grace during this time.

Many new mothers feel frustration during their fourth trimester, wondering why it's suddenly so much harder to keep the house spotless, return to routines they had before getting pregnant, or meet the highly personal or societal standards set for parents.

After labor, it's natural to feel exhausted and burnt out. Your body is in a healing period, and it likely needs more rest than before. When you set goals that account for how you're feeling and what you feel up for, they're less likely to stress you out, and you're more likely to maintain a balanced mindset that allows you to be present for you and your child's needs. Let's face it, in the postpartum period, we're a bit emotionally vulnerable. Setting goals that we can actually achieve means we have more moments to celebrate, helping us build confidence along the way.

A lot of the time in the postpartum period, new mothers feel like they're constantly trying to catch up to what they were once capable of. It's common to miss aspects of pre-parenthood life, like the freedom to be spontaneous or the time to pursue personal hobbies without guilt. These feelings are valid, but dwelling on them usually doesn't offer us any good. At this time, you should focus on embracing the new chapter of life you're entering. You're evolving as a person, not leaving behind pieces of your old self.

I know I've drilled this in already, but likely the most important part of setting goals is ignoring external influences that try to tell you what motherhood should look like. Every parent has a unique path, comparing yours to someone else's is an easy way to experience unnecessary feelings of inadequacy. As long as you continue to do what's best for you and your baby, you're moving in the right direction.

I've got some homework for you, but don't moan and groan yet; I want you to set a goal to pamper yourself. Taking care of yourself is just as important as taking care of your baby, and all it takes are a few small acts of self-care that are incorporated into your daily life. You should do whatever feels best for your emotional and physical well-being, but there are a few activities that are esteemed for their self-care capabilities. Here's a to-do list to get you started:

- Choose 1 book at the beginning of the week and read it in your free time throughout the week.
- Call your best friend or someone who brings you a bit of comfort.
- Buy or make yourself a journal and spend a few minutes each day jotting down your thoughts.
- Take a day off social media (or a week).
- Wake up 15 minutes earlier to have a cup of coffee or tea and set positive intentions for the day.
- Explore a hobby that brings you joy.
- Bake a yummy treat like cookies, a cake, or healthy granola snacks.
- Dive into a DIY project: making a photo album, scrapbooking, or home décor.
- Treat yourself to a mani-pedi, either at a salon or in your home.
- When you don't feel like being a chef after cooking every meal for a week, skip the kitchen and treat yourself to your favorite meal from a nearby restaurant.

These are simple ways to pamper yourself in as little as five minutes, helping you unwind and destress throughout the week. Taking time to care for yourself in any way or seeking support from others is never selfish; it's a healthy way to navigate the post-partum period. It's completely normal to feel overwhelmed as a new mom. Struggling is part of the process, and you're never as alone as you think you are. When you feel like it's all too much, reaching out for help from a support group or therapist can make a world of difference by reminding you of your emotional strength and resilience. Needing support is never a failure. Rather, it means that you're willing to do what's needed to provide the best possible environment for your family.

When we're trying to balance the well-being of ourselves and our family, it can be hard to even think about spending time establishing a connection with a new baby. Regardless, this is an extremely beautiful and meaningful process, and the relationship you build early on will likely affect your family dynamic in the future, too. In the next chapter, we'll explore a variety of ways to create and strengthen your bond with your child.

GIVE OTHER MOMS THE TOOLS THEY NEED TO BOOST THEIR RESILIENCE

At the very start of this book, I shared my own story of new motherhood and the sudden realization that things I used to take for granted—like a good night's sleep—would have to be put on hold. Navigating new motherhood can seem like a constant adaptation to a new identity; one in which the number one priority is your child. But does it have to be a choice between yourself and your child? Your child may now be a separate person but the ties that bond you are as strong as they were when you shared one body. And an infant's well-being is inexorably tied to their mother's health and happiness.

Prioritizing self-care is not just about you; it's about everyone who loves and relies on you. The steps you take now will not only enable you to carry out your tasks as a new mom with greater confidence and joy but also establish a pattern that will stand you in good stead in the long run. Parenting never ends; your child's needs simply change as the years go by. Recognizing your need for sleep, exercise, and mental and emotional balance today will ensure that you never equate love with giving up on *your* definition of a happy life. You can serve as a powerful role model for your child, showing them that listening to their body's needs, letting go of unrealistic expectations, and pursuing their passions make life complete. If you'd like to share the self-care strategies you found within these pages, please take just half a minute to share your opinion of this book.

By leaving a review of this book on Amazon, you'll let others know that making time for self-care is a key component of being a great mother and a fulfilled person.

This unique time in your life is also a great opportunity for you to be a sounding board for others; to share the information you discover and to help other moms value self-care and self-kindness. Simply sharing this book is one way you can be part of a supportive community that is united by the understanding of what it is like to be a new mom.

Scan the QR code below

CHAPTER SIX

CULTIVATING CONNECTION WITH YOUR BABY

"Sometimes, when you pick up your child, you can feel the map of your own bones beneath your hands, or smell the scent of your skin in the nape of his neck. This is the most extraordinary thing about motherhood – finding a piece of yourself separate and apart, that all the same, you could not live without." [1]

JODI PICOULT

The first moment you hold your baby, you feel it; there's an indescribable connection. You're holding something that's essentially a part of yourself, yet it's completely unique from who you are. A mother and her child have a relationship that is unlike any other. That being said, it requires a bit of special care and nurturing to maintain.

Bonding with your baby should be high on your postpartum priority list. It will set the foundation for a loving relationship in the future while supporting your child's cognitive, social, and emotional development. When babies feel a strong and consistent bond with their mothers, they develop a sense of security that develops the infrastructure for their emotional health and stability.

Making efforts to help your baby feel safe and cared for assures them that their needs will be met, giving them the confidence to adapt to the new world around them. Babies rely on someone else to meet their physical and emotional needs, and responding consistently to their cues creates a sense of trust.

Bonding is a crucial element for an infant's healthy brain development. Physical touch, soothing words, and emotional interactions encourage a natural formation of neural connections within the brain that aid in the development of social and cognitive skills. These interactions pave the way for your child to form healthy relationships later in life.[2]

A close bond between a mother and her baby can be a source of regulation when the child struggles with emotional or stress responses. When babies receive touch, sound, or visual cues from their caregivers, their cortisol levels decrease and naturally calm the body so they have an easier time managing stress and developing a sense of resilience. A strengthened relationship with a child can be beneficial to the parents, as well. Mothers who bond consistently release a "love hormone" called oxytocin that promotes feelings of affection and connection. Releasing oxytocin can reduce stress and anxiety to make the postpartum period generally more joyful and fulfilling.

Bonding with your child can even impact their physical health. Babies who experience skin-to-skin contact often sleep better, gain weight consistently, breastfeed easier, and have strengthened immune systems. Skin-to-skin contact is one of the most natural ways to bond with a newborn. One practice, often referred to as "kangaroo care," involves placing your baby directly on your bare chest and allowing them to feel your warmth, hear your heartbeat, and smell your skin. When kangaroo care is initiated in the moments after birth or incorporated into your daily routine, you're likely to experience a wide range of developmental benefits for you and your baby.

Newborns are particularly sensitive to changes in their environment like temperature or activity levels. Engaging in skin-to-skin contact with children stabilizes their body temperature, regulates their breathing, and maintains a steady heart rate. Your body is like a natural incubator to help your child feel warm and cozy. Physical touch can stimulate the baby's natural feeding instincts when you're trying to breastfeed and increase your milk supply, promoting the release of the hormone responsible for milk production (prolactin). When a baby is skin-to-skin with a trusted caregiver, they become more relaxed and less fussy while their breathing becomes more regulated.

According to UNICEF's Baby Friendly Initiative, skin-to-skin contact is beneficial to all mothers and babies, regardless of whether or not they're breastfeeding. Baby Friendly standards encourage skin-to-skin contact for at least an hour immediately following childbirth, if possible. Throughout the postpartum period, this practice should continue to promote emotional bonding and success in breastfeeding.[3] Here's a step-by-step:

1. **Prepare a Comfortable Space:** Find a cozy area where you can sit or recline, such as a hospital bed, a chair, or a couch in your home.
2. **Undress Your Baby:** To maximize skin-to-skin contact, your baby should only be wearing a diaper. If

possible, you should both be bare-chested, covered by a blanket for warmth.

3. **Position Your Baby:** Lay your baby on your bare chest and rest their head against your heart with their tummy directly on your skin. Support their head so their airway remains clear.

4. **Relax:** Take slow, deep breaths to help your body relax. Hold your baby gently and allow them to feel your warmth and hear your heartbeat.

5. **Maintain Contact:** Aim for about an hour of uninterrupted skin-to-skin time, either before bed or while you're watching a show or movie. This is an ideal time to try breastfeeding, as the relaxation often prompts the baby's feeding instincts to kick in.

6. **Repeat:** Try to incorporate this exercise into your routine as often as you can.

Babywearing is another way to build a physical connection between you and your baby. Have you ever seen a mama carry your baby against her body using a carrier or wrap? This is baby-wearing; it's an ancient tradition that's seen a bit of a resurgence in recent years. This popularity is for good reason. Being close to a caregiver offers babies comfort while reducing crying and promoting a sense of security. It makes breastfeeding easier, keeping the baby close to the mother's breast. The positioning also promotes the baby's health and physical development, as keeping them upright can help prevent conditions like reflux.[4]

Mothers who choose to babywear have to maintain an additional set of safety considerations. Caregivers should follow the TICKS rule:

- **Tight:** Make sure your carrier is snug enough to support your baby's spine.
- **In View at All Times:** Keep your baby's face as visible as possible to monitor their well-being.
- **Close Enough to Kiss:** Your baby's head should be close enough to your body that you could easily kiss their forehead.
- **Keep Chin off the Chest:** Your baby's chin should not be tucked into their chest. Keep their head in a comfortable position, making sure they can breathe easily.
- **Supported Back:** The child's back should be in a natural position without slumping or collapsing over.

Your child's comfort relies on several factors. Some carriers are better suited for newborns, while others are designed for older babies or toddlers. Many carriers are more adjustable than others to accommodate different body shapes. Luckily, there are a few types of carriers to choose from:

- **Soft Wrap:** This stretchy fabric wrap provides close, snug support that's ideal for newborns.
- **Woven Wrap:** This offers a more structured option with multiple carrying positions that work for both newborns and toddlers.
- **Ring Sling:** This is a long piece of fabric with rings that make it easy to adjust and take off the carrier at any time.
- **Meh Dai:** This is a hybrid carrier, so it has both straps and a structured panel to carry your baby in multiple positions.

- **Soft Structured Carrier:** This option is easy to use and offers support for older babies with buckles and extra padding.

When you're carrying a newborn, it's easiest to use a soft wrap or sling that allows you to hold them in an upright position. As your child becomes more alert and curious, you can adjust your carrier to a front-facing position so they can engage with their surroundings. Once your baby can sit up without any help, you might transition to back-carrying with a more structured carrier. Generally speaking, you should find a carrier that allows you to be comfortable while offering a safe and rewarding experience.

While we're on the topic of skin-to-skin contact, it's hard to ignore one of the greats: breastfeeding. Nursing promotes a sense of comfort and security in babies as the physical closeness establishes trust. Feeding offers a soothing rhythm to help babies regulate their emotions and build strong emotional foundations. The oxytocin that's released during nursing allows mothers to feel more relaxed and bonded with their babies, preventing postpartum depression and creating a sense of calm. In fact, research has shown breastmilk to be so beneficial for a baby's development that the World Health Organization (WHO), the heavily research-based agency of the United Nations whose purpose is to promote the highest level of health possible internationally, recommends that babies under six months of age be exclusively breastfed, and that they are supplemented with breast milk up to age two or beyond.[5]

That being said, breastfeeding is often easier said than done, and it requires a bit of trial and error. Sometimes, finding comfort in nursing is just a matter of changing positions. Let's explore some of the most common ones:[6]

- **Laid-Back Breastfeeding:** The mother reclines with the baby on her chest as gravity helps the baby latch more naturally.
- **Cradle Hold:** The baby rests their head in the crook of the mother's arm while the body is supported across the lap.
- **Cross-Cradle Hold:** This is just like the cradle hold but the baby's head is supported by the opposite arm to allow more control over the latch.
- **Rugby Ball Hold:** The baby is tucked under the mother's arm with the body facing the side and feet pointing backwards.
- **Side-Lying Position:** Both mother and baby lie on their sides while facing each other.
- **Upright (Koala) Hold:** The baby is seated upright on the mother's lap.
- **Dangle Feeding:** The mother leans over the baby and allows the breast to dangle into the child's mouth. This is especially beneficial for clearing blocked milk ducts.
- **Nursing in a Sling:** A sling or baby carrier allows the mom to nurse hands-free.
- **Double Rugby Hold:** Usually used with twins, this position allows two babies to be tucked under each arm so they can feed simultaneously.
- **Dancer Hand Nursing Position:** This position involves sliding the hand under the breast forward, supporting the breast with three fingers rather than four to form a U-shape with the thumb and forefinger that cradles the baby's chin.

It may take a little while to get it right, but as long as your baby is properly latching onto the breast and you're not experiencing any discomfort, you're on the right track. Be patient—it takes time to master nursing. It's normal to experience difficulty in the early days. Let your baby guide the feeding schedule through cues like rooting or crying; they may be hungrier than expected in the first few weeks. It can be helpful during this time to seek support from experienced loved ones, a lactation consultant at your hospital, or from online resources such as La Leche League International, a nonprofit dedicated to supporting breastfeeding mothers. La Leche League also holds local in-person support meetings which you can find out about by visiting their website.[7]

Experiencing low milk supply or painful feedings can add to the frustration of early parenthood. If breastfeeding is really painful and your baby can't seem to latch on or get enough milk, there are a few possible physical issues that could be in play that can be overcome with the help of your doctor or midwife, such as tongue tie, cleft palate or lips, low milk supply, mastitis infection, or having flat or inverted nipples. Any of these issues can usually be addressed and overcome with the right support, so if any of these apply to you, don't lose hope—reach out! Your doctor or midwife may recommend nursing with a nipple shield, using a breast pump and bottle, using different techniques, or a minor surgical procedure in the case of tongue tie.

What works for one mama may not work for another, so if you're struggling, it's okay to explore alternatives to nursing like formula or mixed feeding! The most important thing is to get your baby fed, and, of course, to preserve your own sanity, which is what this book is all about.

Breast pumping offers an accessible alternative to nursing for those who struggle to get their baby to latch or work during feeding hours. It's a way to provide breast milk to a newborn even when you're not physically able to breastfeed. Using a pump can stimulate milk production and allow other caregivers to feed the baby. There are a few types: a manual breast pump operated by hand, a powered pump that can pump both breasts simultaneously, a wearable breast pump that offers a discreet experience, and a hands-free pump that attaches directly to the breasts and can even be worn with a bra. You can start pumping just a few weeks after birth, and the sessions last about 15-20 minutes.[8] Here's the process:

1. Wash your hands and assemble the pump based on related directions.
2. Center the breast shields over the nipples.
3. Start with a low suction setting and gradually increase it as you go.
4. Pump for 15-20 minutes or until milk production begins to slow down.
5. Store milk in clean, sterile containers and refrigerate or freeze them immediately.

Formula is also commonly used by mothers who struggle to produce milk or simply find convenience in using a breast milk substitute. There are a few types: a cow's milk-based formula that is modified to be digestible for babies, a soy-based formula for babies allergic to cow's milk, and a hydrolyzed formula with broken-down proteins for easier digestion. The process of mixing the formula involves using a sterilized bottle, measuring boiled and cooled water according to the packaging, and shaking the formula into the water until it's completely dissolved.

All feeding options are valid choices for nourishing your baby—the goal is to find what works best for you, your schedule, and your family, and of course, to keep your baby fed and nourished. Some of this process is trial and error, and some of it is listening to yourself and your baby. In the first few months of life, your child will communicate with you using nonverbal cues. Since they can't speak yet, you'll see your baby expressing themselves through crying, sounds, facial expressions, and body movements. Among the most common is crying, which is a direct way for babies to signal when they need something: hunger, tiredness, discomfort, or the need for attention. Some mothers can even distinguish between the different cries. Cries for hunger tend to be rhythmic and repetitive, tired cries may start as whimpering or fussing that escalates with time, discomfort cries tend to be more intense, and pain cries are usually sharp and sudden, followed by pauses of silence or gasps.

Babies also use sounds, like cooing or babbling, to express emotions like contentment or a desire for interaction. Babies use eye contact, smiles, grimaces, and mouth movements to convey emotions, and body movements like movement in arms or legs may signal excitement or distress.

There are several states that you may notice your baby slip into throughout the day, ranging from sleep to wakefulness. In a state of deep sleep, your baby is calm and has slow and regular breathing. They are less likely to wake up than a child in light sleep, who may move around and flutter their eyelids. When they're awake, there are a few phases they may move through. When your baby is on quiet alert, they'll be calm, observant, and ready for interaction. In active alert, your baby may move their arms and legs around. They may appear more engaged but are also much easier to overwhelm or overstimulate.[9]

When your baby is ready for connection, there will be signs. They may make eye contact, smile, coo, or reach toward you, indicating they're ready to engage and are looking for attention or comfort. If they're tired, they may rub their eyes, yawn, fuss, or turn their head away from stimuli. When they're hungry, they may smack their lips, root around, suck on their hands or fingers, or make small fussing sounds. Knowing how to recognize these signs means you can respond promptly and constantly build your connection to each other.

After having a child, there's a lot of information about bonding that comes your way. To make it a bit easier, I've created a chart with some of the basics we've outlined, as well as a few extra ways to bond with your child:

Tip	Description	How-to
Skin-to-Skin Contact	Promotes a sense of emotional bonding and regulates the baby's body temperature, heart rate, and breathing.	Hold your baby on your bare chest for at least an hour daily following birth.
Eye Contact	Strengthens emotional connection and communication between a mother and her baby.	Make eye contact while feeding, cuddling, or playing with your baby to help them feel safe and connected.
Babywearing	Keeps your baby close to promote secure attachment and free up your hands.	Use a carrier or wrap to keep your baby against your body while you carry on with your day.
Responding to Cues	Builds trust and helps the baby feel secure and listened to.	Watch and recognize signals like crying, cooing, and body language. Promptly respond to meet their needs.
Massage and Gentle Touch	Soothes the baby and strengthens your bond through physical connection	Use gentle strokes to massage your baby's skin. Talk or sing softly while you massage them.

Talking, Singing, Reading	Encourages language development and bonding.	Narrate your day to your child or sing lullabies to keep them engaged and connected.
Breastfeeding	Offers intimate time for bonding.	Hold your baby close during feedings and make eye contact.

It's clear that bonding has a significant impact on your baby's emotional and physical development. Each interaction you have with your baby plays a role in forming a secure relationship between the two of you. Your bonding doesn't have to look like everyone else's. Try things until you find what works for you: massaging, talking, or babywearing.

In the following chapter, we'll shift our focus to strategies that will help you introduce your new baby to their older siblings. Having a new child is a transition for every family member, and it makes it substantially easier if you foresee a smooth transition that will inevitably prompt healthy bonding between siblings.

CHAPTER SEVEN

MAKING AND NOURISHING OLDER SIBLING CONNECTIONS

"A sibling bond is like no other; it is a love that withstands time and distance." [1]

RAINBOW ROWELL

Have you seen videos or heard accounts of children who greet their new baby sibling with sweetness and delight from the start? Truthfully, that isn't always how it goes down, and it's perfectly okay if you don't get Instagram-worthy footage of your child smiling down at baby on day one! Despite all my efforts to prepare her, early photos of my eldest daughter with her newborn baby brother show a two-year-old who can best be described as shell-shocked. It was one thing to be told there would be a new baby brother in the house soon, but quite another to be confronted suddenly with a tiny, real-live human who made surprisingly loud and frequent crying sounds at all hours! Now they are BFFs, but it took a lot of time for that friendship to develop.

Sibling relationships are unique. They're like friends we don't have to find, filled with love, shared memories, and an innate understanding of each other's deepest truths. While your children may already have a strong bond, the arrival of a new baby can be overwhelming and may stir up challenging emotions for older siblings. If an older child of yours feels confused, anxious, or even jealous as they adjust to the new dynamics of the family, they're not the only one. Their transition is important, too, and requires a bit of maneuvering to make sure the sibling bond thrives.

When a new baby arrives, their older sibling(s) will react differently based on their developmental stage. Very young children from ages 1 to 2 are still highly dependent on their parents for care, and they might not even fully understand the arrival of a new child. They may experience confusion about the disruption of their usual routine, causing them to become clingy or experience increased tantrums and regressive behaviors. To help them transition into a routine with a newborn, it's important to try to keep the toddler's routine as consistent as possible and involve them in caring for the baby in small ways.[2]

Preschoolers aged 2 to 4 may be more aware of the baby's arrival, but they're also more likely to struggle with feelings of jealousy or compete with the newborn for attention. They have a stronger sense of self, so it's likely that the arrival of a new sibling would make them feel a bit displaced. You're likely to see an increase in regressive behaviors and jealousy, causing mood swings or attention-seeking behavior. To make the transition easier for them, reassure them that they are still loved, important, and involved by including them in tasks like picking out clothes for the newborn and scheduling one-on-one time where you're giving them undivided attention.

School-aged children ages 5 and above tend to show more curiosity and excitement about an incoming sibling, though it may cause them anxiety about their role in the family. Some may express a sense of pride in becoming a "big sibling," while battling potential feelings of frustration when they see the baby getting attention. This is normal. To make it easier, encourage the older sibling to talk about their feelings, reassuring them of their importance in the family along the way.[3]

For a child of any age, it can be extremely helpful to prepare them by explaining what it might look like when the new baby arrives. This means having a conversation with your older children, explaining that babies sleep and cry a lot and that they'll need lots of extra attention. Let them know that this doesn't mean they're less important. Keep these explanations simple, maybe even incorporating storybooks or visual aids about incoming siblings. Encourage them to ask questions about what will change and to share their feelings about being a big sibling.

You don't have to wait until the newborn arrives to introduce them to your older children. During your pregnancy, involve your child by letting them feel the baby kick or helping with preparations. As you're setting up the baby's space, like a nursery, let your children play a part in the tasks and educate them about routines that will become a part of your daily life, like feeding and diaper changes. To help remind them of their unique role in the family, you can give your older children a small gift "from the baby" when they first meet. This will help them associate the new baby with positive feelings that make the whole experience more exciting.

When you bring the baby home for the first time, it's important to try to create a calm and positive environment for your children. As busy as you may be, the priority should be taking care of yourself and your family and staying available to focus on both children. The first step is actively showing excitement about the older sibling's new role as a big sister or brother. They don't have to be besties immediately—just keep it simple and peaceful by letting the sibling interact with the new baby on their own terms, either through gentle touch, light conversation, or watching from a distance. If your child is aged 1-2, give them lots of hugs and cuddles and try to keep them engaged in activities they enjoy when the baby is asleep. Let your older children, aged 2-4, "help" with baby tasks that boost their confidence. When they show interest in the newborn, offer them praise so they know they're on the right track. If your child is a toddler or older, consistently encourage them to be proud of their new role as a big sibling. Assign them small responsibilities, like reading or singing to the baby.

With so much going on in your fourth trimester, it's normal to feel overwhelmed and conflicted about where to focus your attention. You may feel torn between tending to your baby and making sure your older children aren't feeling neglected. Regardless, you still have a duty to understand your child's feelings. If your child seems confused, jealous, or resentful of the new baby, encourage them to express these emotions and let them know that feeling this way is valid. Make a conscious effort to spend quality time with them, even if it's short. Read a book with them, go for a walk, or have a quiet chat before bed to remind them that they're still your priority.

While your children are developing and settling into their roles as siblings, it's important to emphasize that you love them both equally. Avoid comparisons between siblings altogether; these can become sources of resentment that last beyond childhood. Talk to your older child regularly about their feelings and keep them in the loop so they feel included in the new baby's routine. Sometimes, reassuring your child is as simple as involving them in small, manageable activities, like coloring or playing a quick game while caring for the baby. While both (or all) children should feel prioritized, remember: you also need to find time to prioritize yourself. If you're feeling overwhelmed, don't be afraid to seek help and support from family members or friends who may be able to offer extra attention for your older children to maintain a balance.[4]

It helps to begin building the bond between your child and newborn before birth, but after the baby arrives it becomes especially important. Once you take the baby home, it's time to involve your other children in the process. Assign your older child special jobs, like handing you diapers during a change or gently rocking the baby in a stable rocker. All of your children should feel included, like they're an important part of the process. When you're reading a book to your newborn, give your child an opportunity to read some of the pages or roleplay a part of the story. Ask your children to sing to the baby or stay present during feedings to help them feel closer to their new sibling. With so many transitions taking place, it's normal for your daily routine to feel a little interrupted. That being said, your older children still rely on the routine they experience before the arrival of the baby. To maintain a similar sense of balance, continue family rituals like movie nights or outings that make the whole family feel interconnected.

Just like any other part of parenting, learning how to guide the developing relationship between your children and newborn requires a bit of trial and error. There are, however, a few simple and safe tasks that many parents assign to older siblings to keep them involved in the arrival of a new baby. Here are a few tasks you may assign to your children that can help them feel involved and valued in your family dynamic:[5]

- Ask them to fetch diapers or wipes when it's time for a change.
- Encourage them to sing or talk to the baby to show them how it soothes them.
- Let them help with bottle feeding (with supervision!).
- Include your baby when you read books to your baby, like during quiet time or before naps.
- Set your older child up with a cradle or swing so they can gently rock the baby.
- Allow your child to pick out baby clothes for the day or help with dressing tasks.
- Let your older toddler be a "special helper," giving them assignments to put pacifiers or toys back in their respective place.
- Ask your child to help with bath time by passing towels or bath toys to the baby.

If the older siblings feel involved and responsible, they're more likely to have and build off of a positive connection with their new sibling. Each child, depending on their age and development, will respond differently. Regardless of how they're feeling, validating their feelings and providing consistent opportunities to bond with their new siblings means you're contributing to a foundation of positive sibling relationships.

Your family is unique, so you may encounter challenges that feel specific to you or your loved ones. During this time, never let yourself feel too ashamed to seek support from family, friends, or professionals who want to help you navigate the transitions that are occurring. It seems like there are a million things to consider during your fourth trimester. In reality, what's truly important is maintaining a strong relationship with your family, and that includes your partner. In the next chapter, we'll look over what it means to actively rebuild intimacy and tend to your connection with your partner following the arrival of a newborn.

CHAPTER EIGHT

STRENGTHENING PARTNERSHIP AFTER THE BABY

"Equal partnerships are not made in heaven-they are made on earth, one choice at a time, one conversation at a time, one threshold crossing at a time." [1]

BRUCE C. HAFEN

Motherhood is beautiful and impactful, but it's also hard. The arrival of a baby comes with its share of challenges: sleepless nights, new routines, and immense pressure to focus on the baby. Honestly, it's challenging to prioritize the emotional and physical connection you have with your partner in your fourth trimester. You may find that your relationship has been more strained than usual. With so much else on your plate, you have to be intentional with your efforts to rebuild your love and intimacy together.

New mothers and fathers experience significant changes after the birth of a new child. When you have a baby, your family looks a little different, but your support for each other should remain the same. Having positive interactions with a caring partner can alleviate some of the overwhelming pressures that make recovery so challenging. Supportive parents show each other they care by working together on baby-related tasks, making sacrifices so the other can rest, offering to nourish the family, or even just being present to listen and reassure.

Following the birth of a child, many parents experience feelings of isolation or stress that impact the daily recovery process. If you're going into parenting with a partner, they could be a source of emotional support and aid with daily tasks, contributing to a healthier and more balanced postpartum environment.[2]

If you're feeling like your relationship feels a bit off following the birth of a child, you're not the first. Research indicated a considerable drop in both emotional satisfaction and physical pleasure after childbirth, with emotional satisfaction continuing to decline up to 4.5 postpartum.[3] You're both encountering unexpected challenges. This can sometimes make communication feel more transactional and less emotional or passionate. You may have more conversations focused on the logistics of baby care, sleep schedules, and household chores, and fewer conversations about your goals or emotions. Many couples miss the spontaneity of pre-baby life, where they could whip out the door at the thought of a date night and feel carefree while planning the weekend. This is normal. The demands of caring for a newborn add a new layer of time pressure to your relationship, leading to physical and mental exhaustion that makes it difficult to prioritize each other or find time for intimacy.

Remember the baby blues and PPD from earlier? If these are a factor in your fourth trimester, it can be even more difficult to maintain an emotional connection with your partner. It's hard to connect with someone when you don't even have the energy (or time) to connect with yourself. Relationships can become strained when deciding how to divide responsibilities between each other, especially if expectations or preferences differ. Many couples don't even know they have different parenting styles until they have children together. This isn't a reason to panic, but it does add a layer of stress to an already vulnerable dynamic. You may be feeling like you're missing your personal time, or experiencing anxiety about the budget shifts that you're making to account for the new addition.[4]

To sum up: There's a lot going on. It's common for parents to have nurturing their relationship take a backseat, let sex become a distant memory, or even feel as though they love their baby more than they love their partner. These can be pretty sucky feelings, but they're *not* always indications of the end of a relationship. Recognizing the changes that are occurring, in fact, is the first step toward overcoming them together.

Strengthening your romantic relationship following the arrival of a baby doesn't happen on its own. Both parents need to make a conscious effort, even amid the exhaustion and frustration of caring for a newborn. It only takes a few small efforts a day to reconnect. One of the easiest ways to start is by promising each other regular dates, even if you're totally redefining what a "date" can look like. If you're too busy one week to make it out of the house, wait for the baby to sleep to light some candles and enjoy a home-cooked meal together. Healthy partnerships include regular one-on-one time; Make a rule to talk each day, even if it's just for 10 minutes, without interruptions. Don't let conversations about your connection fly under the radar, as these are the discussions that keep your passion afloat.

When you're communicating with your partner during an overwhelming time, remaining open and honest with them can keep you both feeling heard and understood. Regardless of how much we want them to, our partners cannot read our minds. Picking up on each other's signals becomes even more difficult when you're both adjusting to new parenthood roles. This means you have to express your needs clearly, describing the problems you're having and the effect it has on you rather than the person themself. While our feelings can sometimes shift into resentment, trying to focus on crafting "I" statements rather than "you" statements can prevent your conversations from becoming accusatory. You both want to feel supported and appreciated, so try your best to thank your partner when they've helped you with a task or offered a hand when stress is high.

Many of us are battling financial pressures, an added layer of stress to top off our postpartum worries. If you have a partner, tackling these issues together can make the weight on your shoulders a bit lighter.

If you're starting to notice negative patterns emerging in your conversations and interactions, it's best to identify them together, even if it's a bit awkward. You may find that you were missing a perspective that helps you understand the situation more, or that you may need to reach out to a third party, like a professional, to work through deeper-rooted issues.

Need some ideas? Here are a few ways that couples can strengthen their bonds during the postpartum period:[5]

- Pursue each other like it's the first date, surprising your partner with small gestures, notes, or physical affection to reignite the spark.

- Have regular dates, even if they're from home.
- Make a rule to have conversations that aren't about the baby, at least a couple of times a day.
- Cook a meal together or go on a short walk.
- Keep your communications open and clear.
- Attend a therapy session together.

After having a baby, many parents find themselves saying, "Woah, I haven't had sex in how long?" It's common for new parents to have significant shifts in their sexual intimacy following the birth of a child. Whether it's caused by exhaustion, body changes, or the pressures of caring for a baby, many new parents find that their sex drive lowers after birth. Mothers, in particular, go through substantial physical and hormonal shifts that have an impact on their sexual desire or comfortability. Fortunately, it's completely possible to rebuild your intimate relationship, and all it takes is a bit of effort and patience.

Some women simply don't want to have sex or experience fear related to discomfort or pain during intercourse. This is especially common after mothers experience tearing or an episiotomy during birth. If this is the case, it's important to take things slowly and gently, and using plenty of lubrication can make it easier. Breastfeeding adds an additional layer of complexity to intimacy; many women experience vaginal dryness if they're nursing, and their breasts may be tender and leaky. Sex might simply feel different after birth due to changes that occur during physical recovery or an exhausted mindset.

The first step toward rebuilding intimacy in the bedroom is finding time to be together without any children. When you get an opportunity to do so, make a conscious effort to engage with your partner by complimenting them, touching non-erotic parts of their body, and pursuing gentle physical affection that reignites your bond. Being fatigued can make intimacy difficult, reducing both the desire and energy to have sex, so you should try to find time to rest before your quiet moments together. It may feel silly at first, but many couples actually schedule time for intimacy, considering when both partners will feel more relaxed and what works best for their schedules.

If you have specific physical concerns that are holding you back from feeling comfortable with intimacy, it may be helpful to consult with a healthcare provider who can address them.

When you and your partner have a child together, your roles in life have changed, so it's not abnormal for your relationship to change a bit, too. Try to be patient with each other during this time, supporting the conscious efforts you each make to evolve and find a new, comfortable normal. In any relationship, communication is important. In a romantic relationship between two parents, it's everything. If it would benefit your relationship, try incorporating communication exercises into your daily routine to encourage a sense of honesty and openness. Here are a few you might want to try:[6]

- **Extended Eye Contact:** In a quiet space, sit facing each other and set a timer for 3-5 minutes. Maintain eye contact without talking for the entire duration. Observe, without judgment, each other's facial expressions and emotions. Connecting on a non-verbal layer can offer another sense of emotional intimacy.
- **Check-Ins:** Based on your routines, schedule regular check-ins on a daily or weekly basis. During this time, share how you're feeling about the relationship, parenting, or challenges you're facing, and encourage

your partner to do the same. If you're able to truly listen without interruption, this exercise promotes open dialogue and understanding.

- **Three and Three:** When you get a moment alone, share three things you appreciate about your partner and ask them to do the same. Then, both of you share three things that have been challenging. In expressing your gratitude and concerns in a non-confrontational way, you're crafting a sense of appreciation for each other.

- **Validate Each Other:** When you're having conversations, maintain your focus on validating each partner's feelings without judgment. Acknowledge why they feel the way they do by using phrases like, "That must have been difficult for you." These efforts will deepen your empathy for each other and strengthen your emotional connection.

- **Mirroring:** To mirror in a conversation, one partner shares a thought or feeling, and the other "mirrors" it by repeating back what they heard. If you say "I feel overwhelmed with the baby's sleep schedule," your partner would reply with "You feel overwhelmed with the baby's sleep schedule." This is a great way to make sure you both feel acknowledged and avoid miscommunication.

It's normal to face difficulties in your personal relationships following the birth of a child, but you now have the skills and techniques to evolve your connection. Regardless of what your relationship looks like—regular date nights, open discussions, or little gestures of appreciation—if you're finding time to prioritize your partnership, you're keeping your connection alive.

If you're feeling like things are different than they were before, they probably are—you're both evolving! The postpartum time period is an opportunity to work together and seek support from each other, helping you both develop as parents and partners with resilience. Stick around—in the next chapter, we'll explore strategies for balancing work life and motherhood during the postpartum period.

CHAPTER NINE

JUGGLING WORK AND MOTHERHOOD

"When you have children, you have to be fiercely organized to get anything done. I learned that if I don't put myself up on the priority list, somehow my kids will eventually get knocked down on that list." [1]

MICHELLE OBAMA

Michelle Obama's words perfectly encapsulate the feelings of working mothers around the world. Managing work responsibilities and motherhood is like a balancing act in the circus. It's a constant struggle that requires organization, self-care, and prioritization to effectively master. But don't be intimidated—you can do this.

Many mothers have to return to work shortly after giving birth. No matter what your job may look like, returning to work in the post-partum period can be a challenge. Working moms and their children commonly experience separation anxiety, making time apart emotionally difficult for both parties. Working from home has its own set of challenges, especially without adequate childcare. Some mothers may be suffering from postpartum depression or having issues related to their physical recovery process, making the return to work especially difficult. Many of us face financial pressures that add another layer of stress, especially if we're experiencing urgency to return to work. If you're breastfeeding, there may be times when you have to use a pump at work. Pre-planning for pumping in your workspace or office offers another challenge.

When you're raising a newborn, time management is already hard enough. Tack on your work responsibilities, and you've got a recipe for stress. It's definitely not easy to balance work hours with your baby's needs and other household responsibilities. Sometimes it doesn't even seem possible, but you can manage it with a bit of extra planning.[2]

Before returning to work, you can avoid some unwanted stress by planning ahead and building a support system that will ease you back into the workplace. If your children don't already have a caretaker at home when you're at work, arrange childcare for them in advance to give you peace of mind when you're gone. Many mamas choose to do a phased return to work, where they begin with part-time or reduced hours to soften the transition. If you can, reach out to your support network of family, friends, and coworkers who can help you feel less isolated and maybe offer aid when you're unavailable. It can also be beneficial to communicate openly with your employer about your needs, so they can possibly offer you more flexible hours or breaks for pumping. If available to you, take advantage of work-from-home days to stay connected while reducing the shock of making a full return.

It's often easier said than done to set clear boundaries at work. However, without these, the stress of your work and home life can become very conflated. Having open communication with your boss and coworkers may grant you some of the support you need while informing others of what you may need to succeed in the workplace.

If it's all just feeling like too much, try crafting a list of everything you need to do in a day. Then, rank each task based on its necessity and urgency, and prioritize the highest tasks on the list so you're focusing on what's most important. It's normal to be a bit out of practice when you return after maternity leave; you may want to practice your routine before officially returning to work or dedicate some time to upskilling to boost your confidence and make this transition move swiftly. Above all, you should continue to make self-care a priority and be kind and patient with yourself as you adjust.

Achieving balance between your work and your family is not easy, but it becomes a lot harder when you're striving for perfection (hint: you won't find it). Instead, your goal should be prioritizing what's important to you, and showing compassion for yourself and your family. If you can be patient with yourself, it becomes a lot easier to manage time and expectations, thus creating a healthier professional and personal dynamic.

Our conversation about self-care from earlier highlighted the importance of taking time to nurture your mental state in order to be the best mother you can be. This becomes even more relevant when you're trying to balance your role as a mama and your position at a company or workplace.

You're not going to perform perfectly every single day. Life changes, and so do your skills, energy levels, and priorities. Different seasons in your life will require different approaches in order to find balance. You're juggling multiple roles, so it's okay if you don't have all of them completely figured out. Do what you can and be gentle with yourself, even on the bad days. I went back to work expecting to excel, both in my work and my role as mother, and ended up feeling that I had let myself and my children down, all because I didn't meet the rigid expectations I had set. To make the weight of these roles a bit lighter, I eventually realized I needed to delegate tasks at work and home, letting go of the expectation that I could possibly be perfect in every area. If I could speak with that past version of myself knowing what I know now, I would say "Take it easy on yourself Jocelyn! You're doing something really hard, and you need to be kinder to yourself!"

Being a working mom doesn't mean you're selfish, and it doesn't mean you're a failure. You're doing the best you can to support your family and provide for them. When you get to work, be there. Focus on what you have to do to get through the day. This is harder if you work from home, but do what you can to arrange for support during designated working hours so you can focus. When you're home or "off," be present there, as well. Allow yourself to experience a full mental shift to naturally reduce your stress levels and increase satisfaction. When you get a chance, find time for rest. Prioritizing your relaxation is the surest way to avoid burnout and maintain your well-being throughout the week. In your busiest weeks, you may need to make time to rest using time-saving hacks that free up valuable time for your family, like meal prepping or schedule organization.

When you're at work, you should be focused on work. Finding a childcare provider you can trust means that you can stay involved in your tasks without worrying about what's going on at home. Whether this is your partner or a professional childcare consultant, find someone who you know will keep your family in check when you can't be there. If you're parenting with a partner, make sure you're sharing responsibilities as evenly as possible and that you're both on the same page regarding your work-life balance and priorities.

When you have older children in addition to a newborn, there are a few extra considerations you have to make to create a smooth daily routine. Try coordinating naps that align with the schedules of both your toddler and newborn, offering a window of quiet time for you to rest or handle other tasks. If you're on the go and need your hands freed up, wear your younger child in a carrier so you can be hands-on with your toddler. Even in the busiest weeks, make sure you prioritize quality time with your older child, even if it's just for a few minutes during the day. All of your children should feel valued and included. As a reminder, involving your older child in baby care tasks like helping with diaper changes or picking up clutter can grant them a sense of responsibility and connection to their new sibling. The goal is to split your time fairly between your children. Some days, this will be harder to achieve than others. You may feel like your kids are never pleased with your decisions, and that's okay. Give yourself grace as you figure out the right balance to keep everyone (including yourself) as happy and taken care of as possible.

Trust me; I get it. Being a working mama is not easy. We often face an abundance of challenges in balancing our careers with family life, leaving little room for self-care. I know you've heard this before, but if you don't find room for self-care, you won't be as productive or happy as you want to be. Luckily, you can easily incorporate a few self-care strategies into your daily routine to maintain your well-being and prevent burnout. Here are a few you may want to include in your busy schedule:

- Repeat a daily mantra to yourself or use positive affirmations to shift your mindset and keep self-compassion at the forefront.
- Take regular breaks throughout the day to go on a short walk, enjoy a quiet cup of coffee, or engage in a few minutes of mindfulness.
- Maintain focus on your strengths instead of dwelling on weaknesses. Celebrate each little accomplishment, both professional and personal.
- Talk to a friend, family member, or therapist about your feelings. Sometimes, just expressing your concerns can lighten the mental load.
- Do something new every week, like trying a hobby, visiting a new place, or reading a book that keeps your mind engaged and energized.
- Allow yourself 10-15 minutes of "worry time" to address your concerns and negative emotions. After the time is up, let your worries go for the rest of the day.
- Create or join a mommy group full of other working moms who can offer advice or support, share experiences, or help with childcare when needed.
- Schedule a daily 5-minute exercise session to engage in stretching or yoga to boost your energy levels and relieve stress.

I know this is a lot to take in. To make it easier, I've created a box with all of the tips and strategies covered in this chapter:

Transitioning Back to Work	Work-Life-Mom Balance	Managing Other Children	Self-Care Strategies for Moms
Arrange childcare ahead of time.	Consider the season you're in.	Coordinate naps for toddlers and newborns.	Repeat a daily mantra: "I am doing the best I can . . ."
Consider a phased return to work.	Don't try to do it all.	Wear your baby to free up your hands.	Take regular breaks throughout the day.
Build a support network.	Let go of the mom guilt.	Prioritize quality time with older children.	Focus on your strengths, not your weaknesses.
Communicate with your employer.	Wherever you are, be there fully.	Involve your older child in caring for the newborn.	Talk to someone about your feelings.
Use your Keep-in-Touch days.	Look for time-saving hacks.	Split your time fairly.	Do something new every week.
Set clear boundaries.	Find a trusted childcare provider.	Keep everything in perspective.	Set "worry time" to manage concerns.
Prioritize daily tasks.	Talk to your manager about flexibility.		Create a mommy group for support.
Practice routines before returning to work.	Reduce distractions		Schedule a five-minute exercise session daily.
Dedicate time to upskilling.	Don't forget your partner.		

The transition back to work and trying to balance all of your responsibilities can be extremely overwhelming. If done intentionally, however, you can employ certain strategies in your career and family life to protect your well-being and that of your family. You've got the tools to prioritize self-care, set boundaries, and seek support from others, which means you have the power to create a manageable routine that benefits you and your children.

Continue to give yourself grace and celebrate when you've done your best. If you implement the strategies discussed, you'll be able to create space for yourself and nurture your relationships with grace. We're nearly finished; in our final chapter together, we'll cover an in-depth understanding of postpartum self-care, providing you with even more ways to support your health and recovery during the most significant transition of your life.

CHAPTER TEN

LOVING THE NEW YOU

"Love yourself first and everything else falls into line. You really have to love yourself to get anything done in this world." [1]

LUCILLE BALL

Being a mother brings deep joy and fulfillment, but it comes with significant challenges and changes that affect you physically and emotionally. As you move through these transitions and manage the demands of a new child, caring for yourself and prioritizing self-love may be more difficult. But it's more important than ever to help you navigate your new life with resilience and confidence.

Often, mothers want to reject and ignore the negative emotions and struggles they encounter during the postpartum period. It might feel better initially to push these feelings away and pretend there aren't any physical, emotional, or mental changes. They can be overwhelming, but in reality, they offer constant opportunities for deep personal growth. Resisting these changes can leave you stuck, wondering why everything seems to develop while you stay stagnant. If you accept them, you're more likely to rebuild the confidence you need to step into your new identity with grace. While you may not have chosen all of the changes you're experiencing, the postpartum period offers an opportunity to love and appreciate the new version of yourself that motherhood brings.

It's not uncommon to feel like you're going through a particularly hard time after the birth of a child, but keeping a few things in mind can make it easier. Your body has been through an incredible, life-making process, so it's going to look a bit different. These changes are a testament to your strength. If you feel a lot of negativity coming your way, consider your environment; surround yourself with people who are uplifting you and maybe offering support during your postpartum period. Having friends, family, or a support group who truly cares about you can make a big difference to your mental health. Of course, self-care should always be on your mind. Taking care of yourself means getting enough rest and nourishment while finding time to relax and enjoy activities that you love. Reach out to like-minded women who may give you more insight into how they personally achieve their self-care goals.

No matter where you are now, you've come a long way already. Motherhood is full of evolutions, in small ways and large ones. Acknowledging your growth every step of the way can make sure you cultivate a consistently positive mindset. Being a mother doesn't mean your self-discovery is over. Rather, it gives you a chance to rediscover yourself and emerge stronger and more resilient.

The strength of a mother is evident in every step she takes: each of her sleepless nights, hormonal changes, and the juggling act of multiple responsibilities she manages on a daily basis. Her efforts showcase the incredible resilience required to bring life into the world and nurture others (including her own) simultaneously.

Many mothers often don't truly embrace and celebrate the strength they have, but doing so can seriously enhance our well-being. This means acknowledging every achievement and milestone, no matter how average they may feel. When you make it through a sleepless night, spend a little extra time enjoying your pick-me-up in the morning as a reward. After a moment of joy with your child, take a moment to celebrate. After a hard week of balancing work and family night, get your favorite takeout and relax. Every small step you take toward achieving your goals or taking care of yourself and others is worth celebrating.

When we're feeling down on ourselves, we often feel the need to reject any compliments coming our way. When someone praises your efforts as a mother, it's unnecessary and unhelpful to brush this off. Rather, take the time to appreciate it and allow the confidence that comes with this praise to seep in, reinforcing the value of your work.

There may be gaps and barriers in your motherhood journey that are unique to your situation. While they may just seem like burdens, identifying and embracing them means you're doing what you can to grow in the environment you're in. Motherhood doesn't require perfection; it requires growth. Once you really understand your challenges and accept them as they are, you can take steps to move forward from them with strength. Speaking of strengths, identify yours: patience, problem-solving abilities, nurturing skills, or anything else that you enjoy or excel at. Acknowledging these qualities and using them where you can gives you an incredible superpower to carry as a mother.

Acknowledging your strengths verbally can also empower your children by example. Try to show them the importance of resilience, self-love, and confidence through your actions, letting them know that every moment of strength is worth celebrating.

If you're feeling like you've lost a part of yourself or your identity after having a baby, you're not alone. Motherhood changes you, and it often shifts your priorities, routines, and personal goals. You might find yourself so focused on childcare that you don't even think about yourself for days, leaving you feeling like you've lost a part of your old self. This is common, but it doesn't have to be your reality. Change is a natural part of the process, and while you might not have expected it, the person you become after the birth of a child is still someone worth discovering and loving. Coming to this realization is both possible and important for your well-being as a mother.

While it may not feel like your top priority, rediscovering yourself allows you to see your own value beyond being a mother, keeping you grounded and fulfilled. One way to start (and you might not want to hear it) is unplugging from social media. Social networking platforms are often the source of stress and insecurity, and steering clear of them can seriously limit comparison and external pressure. Without all the noise, it becomes much easier to reframe your thoughts and shift from self-doubt to compassion. In your down-time, take a moment to reflect on your values, passions, and goals outside of parenthood. To pinpoint desires you may have mentally set aside, ask yourself the "miracle question": What would you do if you could make one change overnight?

Once you have a good idea of what you want your growth to look like, set new goals that help you focus on it. Maybe you're hoping to return to a hobby you used to love or explore new interests you left behind. When you start to follow through on your goals, remember to prioritize yourself where you can. Step away from your usual responsibilities every once in a while to reconnect with what brings you joy, like reading, painting, or exercising. If you can't pinpoint exactly what you want to do to bring back some passion, try a bunch of things! Taking a walk outside can boost your mood and energy, and trying a new skincare routine can make you feel cared for and more informed. Simply just getting out of the house can help you regain a sense of independence.

When you're feeling particularly down on yourself, try creating a "badass list" of all of your accomplishments, including the tiny ones. This can remind you of all of your strengths and capabilities and offer you tangible evidence to refer back to in your more insecure moments.

Your body might have changed, but that doesn't mean you should stop showing it love. Embrace it as it is now and celebrate it every step of the way. Let yourself fully appreciate each part of your body, verbally or mentally offering yourself supportive words throughout the day. When you just can't seem to find anything you like about yourself, it can help to connect with friends who understand the way you're feeling and offer some support. Remember: comparison is the thief of joy, and that includes comparing your new self to your old one.[2] Motherhood has changed you, and it will continue to. That's okay! You can't go back, but you *can* embrace the new version of yourself. She's just as valuable, vibrant, and worthy of love as she was before.

We're getting close to the end here. You've learned so much about how to acknowledge and take advantage of your own strength and resilience. To hammer in some of these concepts, you may want to consider incorporating daily affirmations into your routine that prepare you for the days ahead and keep your thoughts balanced and positive. To get you started, I've made a list of affirmations that can be repeated to yourself in the morning or throughout the day to offer a confidence boost and keep you on track:

1. I'm doing the best that I can, and that's enough.
2. My body is strong and capable.
3. I deserve the same love and care I offer my baby.
4. I trust myself to consistently make the best decisions for me and my family.
5. I am proud of the person I'm becoming.
6. It's okay to ask for help when I need it.
7. I am patient and compassionate with myself and my family.
8. I embrace the changes that motherhood brings me.
9. I see my value beyond what I achieve in a day.
10. I learn from every mistake.
11. I grow a little every day.
12. I am more than my body.
13. I am enough for my child.
14. I trust my instincts and allow myself to follow my intuition.
15. I am grateful for the path I'm on, even when it gets challenging.
16. I focus on progress, not perfection.
17. The love I have for my child is powerful.
18. I celebrate every victory along the way.
19. I feel confident in my abilities to handle whatever motherhood is bringing my way.
20. I am becoming the best version of myself and the best mother I can be.

I also encourage you to take some time out of your day for self-reflection. A great way to do this is through journaling; I've provided some prompts to guide your writing:

1. What are three qualities of your body you're grateful for? How did these help you bring life into the world?
2. How has motherhood changed how you see yourself?
3. What do you need to feel more supported?
4. How can you show yourself kindness and compassion?
5. What's one way you've surprised yourself, either in your personal life or family life?
6. What's the biggest lesson you've learned about motherhood so far?
7. Name three things that bring you joy outside of parenthood.
8. How can you incorporate more self-care into your daily routine?
9. What strengths have come to light since you've become a mom?
10. How do you currently handle feeling stressed or overwhelmed?
11. What does balance currently look like for you?
12. What would you say to a close friend who was going through what you are right now?
13. How can you celebrate progress?
14. What does self-love currently mean for you?
15. How do you know when you need to ask for help? How can you do it more often?
16. Outside of motherhood, what are your biggest goals? How can you pursue them?
17. What are three things you can do this week to improve your well-being?

18. What emotions do you feel the most since becoming a mother? What prompts them?
19. What are your biggest hurdles at the moment? How can you approach them with a positive mindset?
20. How do you want your children to remember you as a parent?
21. How has your relationship with your partner changed since becoming parents?
22. What hobbies do you miss from before pregnancy? How can you return to them?
23. How can you incorporate mindfulness into your daily interactions?
24. What have you accomplished since becoming a mom?
25. What do you need to let go of to make room for joy?
26. How do you define success as a mother?
27. What's something you'd like to learn about yourself?
28. What do you love most about yourself at this time?
29. What fears do you have about being a mother? How can you release these fears?
30. How can you make more time to connect with your family in meaningful ways?

My goal in designing these prompts and affirmations is to help you reflect, grow, and feel empowered on your motherhood journey. Acknowledging the new version of yourself is the first step of loving it. An empowered mama is one who understands her resilience and uses it to navigate motherhood with confidence and self-compassion. Continue to find ways to celebrate your growth and practice self-care, and you'll start to notice that motherhood comes a bit more naturally.

Take every moment you can to celebrate your strengths; you've undergone an incredible transformation. I can't thank you enough for choosing this book as your companion along the way. It's been a privilege to share my insights with empowered women like you. Keep embracing the radiant mother you've become.

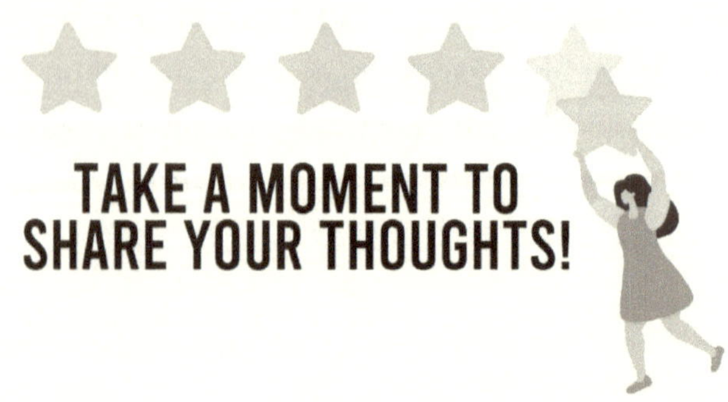

Congratulations on completing your journey through this book! It fills me with joy to think of you and many moms around the world viewing motherhood as a unique opportunity to make new connections. As the years go by, you will remember that one parent who shared a great resource or tool, another who listened to you when you were feeling overwhelmed, or someone who gave you a helping hand when you needed it. This unique time in your life is also a great opportunity for you to be a sounding board for others; to share the information you discover and to help other moms value self-care and self-kindness. Simply sharing this book is one way you can be part of a supportive community that is united by the understanding of what it is like to be a new mom.

Thanks for your help. If you're already feeling more resilient and loving the new you, let others know that they can feel this way, too.

Scan the QR code below

You've come a long way since you started this book.

Take a moment to reflect on everything you've learned and the journey you're currently on, as a mother and as an individual. Motherhood is changing your life, offering new challenges, joys, transformations, and tests. Regardless of what your unique path looks like, you're more than capable of navigating what's coming with resilience and grace.

If there's anything I hope you take away from this book, it's this: to be the best mother you can be, you must take care of yourself first. Continue to practice self-care, set boundaries, and prioritize yourself as you begin to rediscover the version of yourself that motherhood brings out. Taking time for yourself is never selfish—it's the best way to maintain the well-being of yourself and your family.

Since you've picked up this book, you've made a conscious decision to dedicate time and energy to your growth. Your efforts should not go unnoticed, no matter how small they may feel. Each step you take toward shaping a happy and healthy life for your family is a monumental one. If you've made it this far, you're already doing an amazing job. Your first celebration starts now! Give yourself a pat on the back or a reward for everything you've accomplished and learned so far.

I've given you the tools and insights, and the strength has been within you all alone. Now that you know what you have to do, continue applying the strategies I've offered you and adjust them when you feel they could be better suited to your family or personal environment. It won't always be easy, but you are beyond capable of doing your very best, and that is more than enough.

Just as I've shared my story, I'd love to hear yours. If this book has spoken to you, consider leaving a review describing your experience. Your feedback helps me and other mothers who may be looking for the support you found in this book.

Mama, never give up. You've got this!

NOTES

INTRODUCTION

1. Shutterfly Community, "25+ New Mom Quotes And Words Of Encouragement For Mothers," *Shutterfly*, June 8, 2020, https://www.shutterfly.com/ideas/new-mom-quotes/

1. WHY IS POSTPARTUM SELF-CARE IMPORTANT?

1. Leigh Weingus, "55 Inspiring Self-Care Quotes Every Mom Needs In Her Life," *Silk and Sonder*, October 19, 2022, https://www.silkandsonder.com/blogs/news/55-inspiring-self-care-quotes-every-mom-needs-in-her-life
2. WebMD Editorial Contributors, "What Is the Fourth Trimester?" *WebMD*, n.d., https://www.webmd.com/baby/what-is-the-fourth-trimester.
3. Carmen, "Thriving Through the fourth Trimester: Navigating the Challenges of Early Motherhood." *Beautiful Skin By Carmen*, July 5, 2023, https://beautifulskinbycarmen.com/thriving-through-the-4th-trimester-navigating-the-challenges-of-early-motherhood/.
4. "The Importance Postpartum Self Care," *PremamaWellness*, February 22, 2024, https://www.premamawellness.com/blogs/blog/postpartum-self-care.
5. Marcy Crouch, "6 Myths About Your Postpartum Recovery, According to a Physical Therapist," *Healthline*, July 5, 2022, https://www.healthline.com/health/fitness/postpartum-recovery-myths#6-myths-about-postpartum-recovery.
6. "Myths About Postpartum Care," *Ovum Women & Child Speciality Hospital*, Accessed September 2024. https://ovumhospitals.com/blog/myths-about-postpartum-care
7. "Postnatal Rituals from around the World," *The Mindful Birth Group*, April 24, 2023, https://www.themindfulbirthgroup.com/parents/blog/postnatal-rituals-from-around-the-world/.
8. Department of Health & Human Services, "Ayurveda," *Better Health Channel*, accessed September 2024, http://www.betterhealth.vic.gov.au/health/conditionsandtreatments/ayurveda.

2. EMBRACING YOUR BODY'S JOURNEY

1. Kate, "23 Powerful Postpartum Body Quotes," *Mom with Anxiety,* 2024, https://momwithanxiety.com/postpartum-body-quotes/
2. "Pregnancy: Physical Changes After Delivery," *Cleveland Clinic,* last modified January 1, 2018, https://my.clevelandclinic.org/health/articles/9682-pregnancy-physical-changes-after-delivery.
3. "Body Changes When You Have a New Baby," *Tommy's,* last modified March 11, 2021, https://www.tommys.org/pregnancy-information/after-birth/body-changes-when-you-have-new-baby.
4. "Hair loss in new moms," *American Academy of Dermatology Association,* n.d., https://www.aad.org/public/diseases/hair-loss/insider/new-moms#:~:text=Many%20new%20moms%20see%20noticeable,caused%20by%20falling%20estrogen%20levels.
5. "Care for Your Nursing Breasts," *American Pregnancy Association,* accessed September 2024, https://americanpregnancy.org/healthy-pregnancy/breastfeeding/care-for-your-nursing-breasts/.
6. Sara Lindberg, "Breasts After Breastfeeding: How They Change and What You Can Do," *Healthline,* July 24, 2020, https://www.healthline.com/health/breastfeeding/breasts-after-breastfeeding#what-you-can-do.
7. Adam Smith, "Comparison is the death of joy," *Adam Kirk Smith* (blog,) October 8, 2017, https://asmithblog.com/comparison-death-joy/

3. ESSENTIALS FOR NURTURERS TO FUEL THEIR POSTPARTUM RECOVERY

1. Leigh Weingus, "55 Inspiring Self-Care Quotes Every Mom Needs In Her Life," *Silk and Sonder,* October 19, 2022, https://www.silkandsonder.com/blogs/news/55-inspiring-self-care-quotes-every-mom-needs-in-her-life
2. Mary Chong and Marjorelee Colega, "Postpartum Nurtrition – Your Road to Recovery," *Health Hub,* last modified November 15, 2022, https://www.healthhub.sg/live-healthy/postpartum-nutrition-your-road-to-recovery.
3. Sara Lindberg, "Postpartum Diet Plan: Tips for Healthy Eating After Giving Birth," *Healthline,* July 31, 2020, https://www.healthline.com/health/postpartum-diet#weekly-meal-plan.
4. "Maternal Diet and Breastfeeding," *Centers for Disease Control and Prevention,* accessed 2024. https://www.cdc.gov/breastfeeding-special-circumstances/hcp/diet-micronutrients/maternal-diet.html#:~:text=This%20means%20approximately%202%2C000%20to,not%20pregnant%20and%20not%20breastfeeding.
5. Sara Lindberg, "How to Find Relief from Postpartum Insomnia," *Healthline,*

September 26, 2022, https://www.healthline.com/health/postpartum-insom nia#bottom-line.

6. "7 Tips for Prioritizing Sleep During the Postpartum Period," *Sweet Child O'Mine,* April 3, 2022, https://sweetchildbirth.com/2022/04/03/sleep-during-the-postpartum-period/.

7. "Safe return to exercise after pregnancy," *Pregnancy: Birth & Baby,* accessed September 2024, https://www.pregnancybirthbaby.org.au/safe-return-to-exercise-after-pregnancy#:~:text=Regular%20exercise%20after%20you%27ve,pre vious%20level%20of%20physical%20activity.

8. Mayo Clinic Staff, "Labor and Delivery, Postpartum Care," *Mayo Clinic,* March 13, 2024, https://www.mayoclinic.org/healthy-lifestyle/labor-and-delivery/in-depth/exercise-after-pregnancy/art-20044596.

4. NAVIGATING BABY BLUES AND POSTPARTUM DEPRESSION

1. Kate, "23 Powerful Postpartum Body Quotes," *Mom with Anxiety,* 2024, https://momwithanxiety.com/postpartum-body-quotes/

2. Lizabeth A. Kopp and Judi R. Gedaris, "What Happens to Your Hormones After Birth?" *Hackensack Meridian Health,* March 2, 2023, https://www. hackensackmeridianhealth.org/en/healthu/2023/03/02/what-happens-to-your-hormones-after-birth.

3. Alyssa Sybertz, "How Do Hormones Change Postpartum?" *HealthCentral,* July 9, 2024, https://www.healthcentral.com/womens-health/postpartum-hormones.

4. Lauren Osborne and Lindsay R. Standeven, "Baby Blues and Postpartum Depression: Mood Disorders and Pregnancy," *John Hopkins Medicine,* accessed September 2024, https://www.hopkinsmedicine.org/health/well-ness-and-prevention/postpartum-mood-disorders-what-new-moms-need-to-know.

5. Sarah Bradley, "What Are the Baby Blues and How Long Do They Last?" *Healthline,* May 7, 2020, https://www.healthline.com/health/baby-blues#symptoms.

6. Mayo Clinic Staff, "Postpartum Depression," *Mayo Clinic,* November 24, 2022, https://www.mayoclinic.org/diseases-conditions/postpartum-depres sion/symptoms-causes/syc-20376617.

7. Debra Fulghum Bruce, "Postpartum Depression," *WebMD,* August 23, 2022, https://www.webmd.com/depression/postpartum-depression.

8. Mindful Staff, "What is Mindfulness?" *Mindful,* July 8, 2020, https://www. mindful.org/what-is-mindfulness/.

9. Edith Gettes, "Composing a Moment: Mindfulness Techniques in Post-partum Mood Disorders," *Postpartum Support International,* August 5, 2016, https://www.postpartum.net/mindfulness/.

10. Tamara Barak Aparton, "The Best Postpartum Yoga Routine," *Parents,* December 4, 2023, https://www.parents.com/pregnancy/my-body/postpartum/5-yoga-poses-for-postpartum-abs/.

5. SELF-CARE PRACTICES FOR POSTPARTUM MOMS

1. Kristi Yeh, "23 Self-Care Quotes for Parents," *Parent Self Care,* April 22, 2024, https://parentselfcare.com/blog/23-self-care-quotes-for-parents
2. BetterHelp Editorial Team, "Why Does Self-Care for Mothers Matter for Mental Health?" *BetterHelp,* last modified September 25, 2024, https://www.betterhelp.com/advice/mindfulness/why-self-care-is-important-for-mothers/.
3. Kelsey Atkinson, "The Importance of Setting Boundaries as a New Parent: Protecting Your Mental Health and Well-Being," *Kelsey Atkinson Counseling & Sleep Consulting,* accessed September 2024, https://www.kelseyatkinson-counselling.com/sleep-tips/the-importance-of-setting-boundaries-as-a-new-parent-protecting-your-mental-health-and-well-being.
4. Kristin Neff, "Self-Compassion," *Self-Compassion.org,* accessed September 2024, https://self-compassion.org/what-is-self-compassion/.
5. Natalie Bacon, "How to Practice Self Compassion as a Mom," *Mom On Purpose,* February 14, 2024, https://momonpurpose.com/how-to-practice-self-compassion-as-a-mom/.
6. Sarah Barkley, "Self Expectations: 7 Suggestions for Setting Realistic Expectations," *PsychCentral,* October 28, 2022, https://psychcentral.com/health/suggestions-for-setting-realistic-expectations-with-yourself.

6. CULTIVATING CONNECTION WITH YOUR BABY

1. Jessica Vacco-Bolanos, "Relax, Enjoy and Breathe in That New Baby Smell—Here Are 150 New Mom Quotes," *Parade,* May 12, 2024, https://parade.com/1098145/jessicavacco/new-mom-quotes/
2. "Bonding with Your Baby," *Pregnancy Birth & Baby,* accessed September 2024, https://www.pregnancybirthbaby.org.au/bonding-with-your-baby#:~:text=A%20bond%20between%20a%20baby,cells%20in%20your%20baby%27s%20brain.
3. Baby Friendly Initiative, "Skin-to-Skin Contact," *UNICEF United Kingdom,* accessed September 2024, https://www.unicef.org.uk/babyfriendly/baby-friendly-resources/implementing-standards-resources/skin-to-skin-contact/.
4. WebMD Editorial Contributor, "Baby Wearing: What Is It?" *WebMD,* April 15, 2023, https://www.webmd.com/baby/what-is-baby-wearing.
5. "Breastfeeding," World Health Organization, accessed October 2024, https://www.who.int/health-topics/breastfeeding#tab=tab_1
6. "11 Different Breastfeeding Positions," *Medela,* accessed September 2024,

https://www.medela.com/en/breastfeeding-pumping/articles/breastfeeding-tips/11-different-breastfeeding-positions.

7. "Find a La Leche League Leader or Group Near You," La Leche League International, accessed October 2024, https://llli.org/get-support/

8. Healthwise Staff , "Breastfeeding: How to Use a Breast Pump," *HealthLink British Columbia*, November 9, 2022, https://www.healthlinkbc.ca/health-topics/breastfeeding-how-use-breast-pump.

9. "Understanding What Your Baby Wants or Needs," *Plunket*, accessed September 2024, https://www.plunket.org.nz/child-development/communication/communication-newborn-3-months/understanding-what-your-baby-wants-or-needs/#:~:text=To%20help%20you%20figure%20out,to%20be%20needing%20or%20wanting.

7. MAKING AND NOURISHING OLDER SIBLING CONNECTIONS

1. The Blinkist Team, "15 Heartwarming Sibling Quotes That Will Make You Appreciate Your Brothers and Sisters," *Blinkist*, July 31, 2023, https://www.blinkist.com/magazine/posts/15-heartwarming-sibling-quotes-will-make-appreciate-brothers-sisters?utm_source=cpp

2. "How to Prepare Your Older Children for a New Baby," *HealthyChildren.org*, April 10, 2019, https://www.healthychildren.org/English/ages-stages/prenatal/Pages/Preparing-Your-Family-for-a-New-Baby.aspx#:~:text=Set%20aside%20special%20time%20for,when%20you%20feed%20the%20baby.

3. Kelsey Klaas, "How Older Siblings May React to a New Baby," *Mayo Clinic Press*, July 28, 2022, https://mcpress.mayoclinic.org/parenting/how-older-siblings-may-react-to-a-new-baby/#:~:text=School%2Dage%20children%20%E2%80%94%20Children%20age,child%20about%20your%20newborn%27s%20needs.

4. "How to Help Your First Child Not Feel Neglected with a New Baby," *American SPCC*, October 7, 2019, https://americanspcc.org/how-to-help-your-first-child-not-feel-neglected-with-a-new-baby/#:~:text=Once%20the%20baby%20is%20born,newest%20member%20of%20the%20family.

5. "10 Ways an Older Sibling Can Help with New Baby," *Baby Brezza*, accessed September 2024, https://babybrezza.com/blogs/news/10-ways-an-older-sibling-can-help-with-new-baby.

8. STRENGTHENING PARTNERSHIP AFTER THE BABY

1. "Partnership Quotes," *AZ Quotes*, accessed 2024. https://www.azquotes.com/quotes/topics/partnership.html

2. "New Dads & Partners: How Your Involvement Matters," *HealthyChildren.org*, June 13, 2024, https://www.healthychildren.org/English/ages-stages/baby/Pages/A-Special-Message-to-Fathers.aspx.

3. Hannah Woolhouse, Ellie McDonald, and Stephanie Brown, "Changes to Sexual and intimate Relationships in the Postnatal Period: Women's Experiences with Health Professionals," *Australian Journal of Primary Health* 20, no. 3 (2014): 298–304, https://doi.org/10.1071/PY13001.

4. Elena Mauer, "A Look at Why Relationships Change After You Have a Baby," *Healthline*, December 3, 2019, https://www.healthline.com/health/parenting/relationship-changes-after-baby#New-baby,-new-you,-new-everything-.

5. Jancee Dunn, "Boost Your Bond—How to Stay Connected to Your Spouse after You Have Kids," *Motherly*, August 30, 2017, https://www.mother.ly/life/boost-your-bondhow-to-stay-connected-to-your-spouse-after-you-have-kids/.

6. Zoë O'Connor, "17 Communication Exercises for Couples," *Paired*, March 1, 2024, https://www.paired.com/articles/communication-exercises-for-couples.

9. JUGGLING WORK AND MOTHERHOOD

1. Nadine Stille, "55 uplifting and powerful working mom quotes to rock your world," *Nadine Stille*, 2024. https://nadinestille.com/article/55-uplifting-and-powerful-working-mom-quotes-to-rock-your-world

2. Paul Brown, "11 Top Tips for Returning to Work Postpartum," *FDM Group*, December 5, 2023, https://www.fdmgroup.com/news-insights/returning-to-work-postpartum/#:~:text=Besides%20a%20range%20of%20physical,or%20dealing%20with%20sleepless%20nights.

10. LOVING THE NEW YOU

1. Amanda N, "70 Inspirational Mom Self Care Quotes For Awesome Moms.," *Mumtastic Life*, May 6, 2022., https://mumtasticlife.com/70-inspirational-mom-self-care-quotes-for-awesome-moms/

2. "Quote Origin: Comparison is the Thief of Joy," *Quote Investigator*, February 6, 2021. https://quoteinvestigator.com/2021/02/06/thief-of-joy/

www.ingramcontent.com/pod-product-compliance
Lightning Source LLC
Chambersburg PA
CBHW051310250726
48656CB00004B/1585